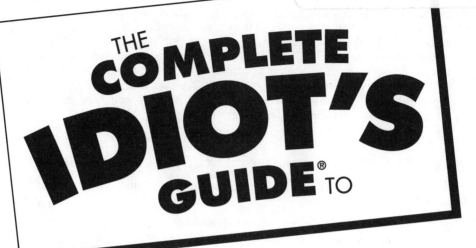

Homeopathy

by David Sollars

alpha
books

201 West 103rd Street
Indianapolis, IN 46290

A Pearson Education Company

Copyright © 2001 by David Sollars

Permission granted by The Institute of Classical Homeopathy (1997) for material used.

Permission granted by Hahnemann Laboratories, Inc., for material used.

THE COMPLETE IDIOT'S GUIDE TO and Design are registered trademarks of Pearson Education.

International Standard Book Number: 0-02-864003-9
Library of Congress Catalog Card Number: Available upon request.

03   02   01   8 7 6 5 4 3 2 1

Interpretation of the printing code: The rightmost number of the first series of numbers is the year of the book's printing; the rightmost number of the second series of numbers is the number of the book's printing. For example, a printing code of 01-1 shows that the first printing occurred in 2001.

Printed in the United States of America

Publisher
Marie Butler-Knight

Product Manager
Phil Kitchel

Managing Editor
Jennifer Chisholm

Senior Acquisitions Editor
Renee Wilmeth

Development Editor
Joan D. Paterson

Technical Reviewer
Savitri Clarke

Production Editor
Billy Fields

Copy Editor
Faren Bachelis

Illustrator
Jody P. Schaeffer

Cover Designers
Mike Freeland
Kevin Spear

Book Designers
Scott Cook and Amy Adams of DesignLab

Indexer
Tonya Heard

Layout/Proofreading
Svetlana Dominguez
Liz Patterson
Gloria Schurick

Contents at a Glance

Contents

Foreword

It's quite fortunate that this book is written by an individual who exemplifies both aspects of the new paradigm that is homeopathic medicine. Homeopathy is an art and a science. The medical practitioner of the new millennium will combine a grasp of the scientific concepts of homeopathy and medicine but will, as important, practice from the heart and spirit. Both David Sollars and his technical editor, Savitri Clarke, are special practitioners—immediately you see that they have big hearts, gentle spirits, good humor, and critical astuteness—all at the same time.

These special scientific and spiritual qualities also relate to the application and even preparation of homeopathic medicines. They seem like incongruent opposites but in reality they are not exclusive to each other. The seeming paradoxes that are homeopathy, is one of the reasons for the difficulty in explaining some of homeopathy's concepts and processes. This book tackles this challenge and successfully allows you, the reader, to grasp the fundamentals of homeopathy. After reading this book you will have an excellent fundamental knowledge of homeopathy and what a homeopath does.

Homeopathy has a profound ability to cure even very serious diseases. We, as homeopathic practitioners, have an opportunity to see dramatic changes in individuals that we treat. As a practitioner and teacher, over the 24 years of practice I have seen that homeopathy can not only cure disease but facilitate a freedom from suffering on all levels—physical, emotional, and mental. Can you imagine a medicine that could treat the whole person more effectively? This emphasis on the inter-relationship of all functions in the body, psyche, and spirit make homeopathy one of the few "holistic" and truly effective medicines.

By presenting in this book, in a well-organized fashion, good-cured cases of various kinds of patients with various kinds of ailments or diseases, you get a sense of the awesome power of well-applied homeopathy. This book offers introductory guidelines including precautionary information about certain conditions for you to start using or participating in homeopathic medicine for yourself or your family. It also brings the reality of how homeopathy can work in the context of a health team of practitioners or on its own. The book gives you references to resources and practitioners for more complex and advanced treatment and learning.

Even though your health and the health of your relatives is a serious matter, the author has done a great job of making the presentation of all this information fun and absorbing. This makes it all the more easy to understand. I encourage you to read this book to enjoy all that is homeopathic medicine and what it can offer you and mankind.

—Louis Klein

Louis Klein is a world-class senior practitioner of homeopathy who has been instrumental in setting educational and professional standards for homeopaths. Lou practices in Vancouver, British Columbia, with Vancouver Homeopathic Associates.

Introduction

Those of us who use the medical art of homeopathy, whether it's in a medical practice or on family members at home, have inherited an enormous body of literature whose thoroughness and insight reflect upon its dedicated healers. Two centuries of homeopathy have been underscored by a selfless sense of compassion, combined with a determined search for the best help we can give our bodies to heal. Although the word *homeopathy* in the general public has become synonymous with natural, non-toxic, safe treatments, I believe a fuller understanding of its potential is needed for this complete healing system's value to be realized. Continued education for our homeopathic practitioners and the general public is an essential part of the awareness that can lead to more accurate prescribing that will result in health and satisfaction for all patients.

Homeopathic medicines hold much promise for a world that is still plagued by chronic diseases. I was certainly doubtful of the seemingly miraculous results that I heard of from homeopaths until I began to understand how the body heals in a homeopathic way. I began to see the benefits of homeopathy reflected in the growing joy and health of my patients. I've included many patients' stories in this book so that you can get a glimpse of the process of choosing a remedy and have a better understanding of how homeopathy works. I envision a time when patients can receive the best coordinated care possible drawn from the most effective arenas of medicine. I have written this book to help practitioners and patients evolve a better medical service for the needs of the world that still strives for health and well-being.

How to Use This Book

For your convenience, this book is divided into five parts. You can search through the conditions that you need immediate relief from, or browse sections for a friend. Since the best homeopathic medicine is based on individual evaluation and diagnosis, the explanations and advice given in this book are meant to be instructive, but do not replace the proper care given by a qualified practitioner. Statistically, most patients do not tell their conventional physicians that they are using homeopathic medicine. I encourage you to read these chapters, which include information in both therapies, so that you can be better informed about your condition and choices. Talk with your doctor and your health-care providers.

Part 1, "Homeopathy ... When Less Is Best," demystifies the basic foundation and theories of homeopathy. In easy-to-read language, it provides the latest research, along with the history of homeopathy in the United States and abroad. You'll learn how homeopathic medicines are researched and manufactured, and where they come from. I'll introduce you to the pioneers of homeopathy and teach you about their critics and supporters.

Parts 2, "Symptoms and Simillimums," 3, "Putting Out Fires," and 4, "Healing with Homeopathy," cover a sampling of conditions for which homeopathy is helpful. Through patients' stories, you'll see what your first visit to the homeopath is like, learn about the process of getting well, and understand the reason your homeopath chooses a particular remedy for you.

Part 5, "Integration and Participation," will help you to understand how to choose and work with a qualified homeopath for better health. We'll discuss how to recognize when you're getting better, the do's and don'ts of treatment, and your role in maintaining your well-being.

At the end of the book, I've included a glossary of terms that are used in homeopathy, as well as a host of resources that will allow you to expand your knowledge of homeopathy and find a qualified practitioner should the need arise. I hope you enjoy this book and that it opens new possibilities for health and freedom for you and your family.

Bonus Boxes for Better Understanding

Throughout the book I've provided boxes that contain valuable tips for treatment and further understanding of homeopathy.

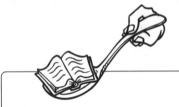

Dose of Info

Easy-to-read definitions of terms and word origins.

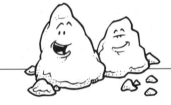

Natural Nuggets

Tips and how-to's for getting better results from your self-care and health care.

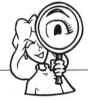

Curious Clues

Case highlights describing symptoms that help homeopaths prescribe the right remedy.

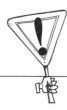

Caution Keeper

Pay close attention to these warnings and potential hazards to your health.

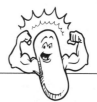

Potent Pellets

Tidbits of news for your review that will deepen your understanding of homeopathy.

Acknowledgments

We would not even be having a conversation about homeopathy if it were not for the curiosity and commitment of Samuel Hahnemann and the many men and women who saw the potential of this medical art and acted on it. Their frustration with the "status quo" was transformed by ingenuity and open-mindedness in creating a new medical model for health and well-being. The tremendous efforts of time and energy needed to research, record, teach, and guide the homeopathic profession through its roller coaster ride of popularity is a debt we can only hope to repay by using homeopathy in the most responsible way.

I am continually impressed by the quality of practitioners that homeopathic medicine attracts to its ranks. Savitri Clarke is a friend and an excellent homeopath who has lent her considerable talents to this book through submitting some of her patient cases and the valuable contributions of ideas that made this book accurate and informative. I have a deep admiration for her abilities and had found her a joy to work with. Karen A. Komisar, D.V.M., a homeopathic veterinarian, made it possible to give you reliable information about the care of your faithful pets. She is the president of the Academy of Veterinary Homeopathy (2000–2001) and continues to be an innovator and educator in this field. Pam Herring is a dedicated and conscientious homeopath who allowed me to share her cases to help illustrate the healing potential of homeopathy.

The following individuals and organizations were eager to help me by contributing advice, discussions, pictures, or articles. My thanks go out to Michael Quinn of Hahnemann Laboratories; Miranda Castro at Kent Homeopathic Assoc.; The National Center for Homeopathy; The North American Society of Homeopathy; Dr. Bill Gray, author of *Homeopathy: Science or Myth;* The European Center for Classical Homeopathy; and Nicola Henriques of The Institute of Classical Homeopathy.

I want to acknowledge the influence and inspiration I have received from my homeopathic teachers, fellow practitioners, and my patients who honor me with the continued trust of caring for them and their families.

And thanks to all the great editors at Alpha Books—Renee Wilmeth, Joan Paterson, Faren Bachelis, and Billy Fields. Your skill and guidance shepherded this project from an idea through all the complexities of publishing a book. You are all expert in your craft.

I want to dedicate this book to my wife Diane who deserves special recognition for her active role in helping me to see this book through to completion. She has worked with me from the beginning on research, format, inputting text, and as a great editor. She shouldered the responsibilities of running our home, caring for our children, and working full-time while this book was being written. I am blessed to have such a talented and generous partner in life.

Special Thanks to the Technical Reviewer

The Complete Idiot's Guide to Homeopathy was reviewed by an expert who double-checked the accuracy of what you'll learn here, to help us ensure that this book gives you everything you need to know about homeopathy. Special thanks are extended to Savitri Clarke, Lic. Ac., C.C.H.

Trademarks

All terms mentioned in this book that are known to be or are suspected of being trademarks or service marks have been appropriately capitalized. Alpha Books and Pearson Education cannot attest to the accuracy of this information. Use of a term in this book should not be regarded as affecting the validity of any trademark or service mark.

Part 1

Homeopathy ...
When Less Is Best

Homeopathy has a colorful and evolving history in medicine, research, and politics. Although the practice of homeopathy has become popular again in this country, the use of this nontoxic and relatively inexpensive medicine has continued to grow world-wide over the last 200 years.

You'll learn what homeopathy is and how it works, both from the latest research to the feelings and sensations that show a trained practitioner you're healing. I'll demystify the manufacturing process, giving you an inside look into how homeopathic remedies are prepared and the standards that ensure your confidence and safety. You'll discover how a plant goes from an herb to a homeopathic remedy. You'll learn what role the FDA plays in standardizing these potent pellets, and how in this country, homeopathy led the way toward organizing the medical community in the United States.

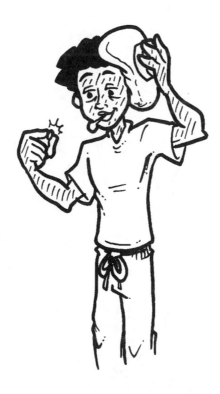

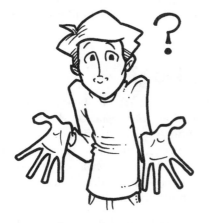

Chapter 1

What Is Homeopathy and How Does It Work?

In This Chapter

➤ Demystify the meaning of homeopathy

➤ Understand how homeopathic medicines help to heal your body

➤ Review the latest scientific studies on how homeopathy works

➤ Discover how water can be made into a powerful healing partner

➤ Learn how homeopathy may be the answer to chronic illness

Chronic illness is a major reason that a great many of us do not live our lives to the fullest. Homeopathic medicines were created to stop the cycle of chronic complaints while restoring health and well-being.

More than 50,000 doctors around the world use homeopathic medicines, according to the Hahnemann Laboratory, one of the leading manufacturers of homeopathic medicines, located in San Rafael, California. A growing number of licensed health practitioners, professional healers, and moms are using homeopathic medicines to aid in the health and healing of their patients and families. However, while more people are examining the merits of homeopathy, others are questioning the effectiveness of its healing properties.

In this chapter you will discover that homeopathic medicines are designed to jump-start your own body's healing abilities. We will examine some revolutionary new scientific findings about homeopathy, which will help explain the healing potential that homeopathic practitioners have observed for more than two centuries. We begin our journey together by delving into a medical art that I believe may hold great benefits for you.

Homeopathy: The Hair of the Dog?

Homeopathic medicines, or remedies as they are often referred to, belong to a pharmaceutical system that prescribes extremely small doses of substances derived mainly from the plant, mineral, and animal kingdoms. Homeopathic medicines are prescribed based on the discovery that whatever symptoms a substance causes in large doses (toxic effect) will help to rally the body's natural healing response in people with similar symptoms or suffering when given in very minute doses (nontoxic). Homeopathic medicines help boost your body's ability to heal itself.

Let's take a quick look at a common example of how this nontoxic approach differs from what you may be used to doing for your health. When you have trouble sleeping and it becomes a growing concern, conventional medicine offers a drug that brings on forced artificial sleep. This may involve the use of large or regular doses of the drug, which can sometimes cause side effects or become addictive. The homeopathic method involves giving you a minute dose of a substance that has been incredibly diluted so that there is no danger of unwanted chemical reactions, typically called side effects. Since your own body is doing all the healing work, you can't get addicted to the substance.

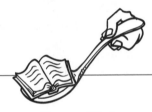

Dose of Info

The word **homeopathy** comes from the Greek words *homos* (similar) and *pathos* (suffering). The way you experience sickness and health are the key characteristics your homeopath will focus on for choosing an accurate homeopathic medicine. You may have the same general diagnostic name—headache, arthritis, or anxiety. Proper homeopathic prescribing targets symptoms and feelings unique to you while finding a substance that matches your own experiences or "similar suffering."

Homeopathic remedies, or homeopathics, are specially prepared with minute amounts of an active ingredient that do not cause side effects or become chemically addictive. In fact, the practice of homeopathy recommends discontinuing remedies when your own system functions properly. Whatever remedy is chosen, it will be based on the entire person's health to ensure an accurate homeopathic prescription that stimulates your body to self-heal in many ways, including better sleep, for example.

Homeopathy gained its initial popularity in Europe and the United States during the 1800s because of its successful nontoxic treatment of infectious epidemics that savaged both continents. During that time, medical cures were often as dangerous as the diseases. People who kept getting sick despite their own best efforts were looking for other health-care options. Sound familiar?

The Rise of Medical Options

The last decade has produced an unprecedented increase in the use of what is termed *complementary alternative medicine (CAM)* or integrative medicine. This definition includes many of the nonconventional therapies such as acupuncture, chiropractic, and massage as well as the use of vitamins and herbs. The growing popularity is illustrated by the increased coverage on television, the Internet, newspapers, and magazine covers devoted to the old and new forms of healing. An article released in the November 11, 1998, issue of the *Journal of the American Medical Association* titled "Trends in Alternative Medicine Use in the United States From 1980–97" shocked many health watchers by revealing that 628,855,000 visits had been made to alternative care providers in 1997 alone, while only 427,120,000 visits were made to primary care providers.

The search for alternate care providers seems to be centered around the age-old desire to feel better and get on with life. According to the *Guide of Coverage of Complementary and Alternative Medicine, 2000 Edition*, the main reasons for using alternative medicines include ...

➤ Preventing illness or injuries (30 percent).

➤ Contributing to wellness (44 percent).

➤ Addressing specific health problems (79 percent), such as back pain (36 percent), headaches (18 percent), and anxiety and emotional problems (13 percent).

As you will learn, homeopathy has been practiced widely throughout much of Europe, India, and other countries during its 200 years of continued evaluation and refinement. Recently, in the United States, homeopathy has been steadily gaining popularity and acceptance after following a boom and bust relationship that will be described in later chapters.

A national survey conducted by Landmark Healthcare in November 1998 revealed that 61 percent of those surveyed were very or somewhat likely to use homeopathy. According to the publication *The State of Healthcare in America*, published in 1998, there were an estimated 3,000 homeopaths, whose number included 500 medical doctors. They estimated homeopathy to be a $200 million-a-year business. What this tells me is that Americans are still not completely satisfied with their current

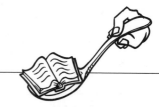

Dose of Info

Complementary alternative medicine (CAM) includes nonconventional therapies such as homeopathy, accupuncture, and massage. The National Institutes of Health (NIH) created the Office of Alternative Medicines (OAM) to coordinate the growing number of funded studies to investigate the efficacy of many CAM therapies. This branch recently formed its own separate organization, the National Center for Complementary Alternative Medicine (NCCAM), to more efficiently handle this rapidly expanding field.

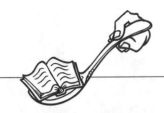

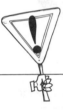

state of health and are looking to include other options that may assist in more complete healing from chronic complaints and help them live with a sense of overall well-being.

Chronic Illness: The Unwelcome Guest

I am clearly reminded in my clinical practice that our society still bears a heavy burden under the weight of *chronic diseases.* Many families struggle through the emotional and financial burdens of conditions that, despite continued treatments, do not fully heal. Others are trapped in a cycle of prolonged drug use that they may vocally rebel against, but often rely on these medical agents for even the most basic functions of life.

We may not be gaining on the eradication of illness as illustrated by the sharp rise of asthma since 1980. Today, according to *The Robert Wood Johnson Foundation's 1999 Annual Report,* there are 17 million Americans who suffer from asthma, 5 million of whom are children. The deaths attributed to asthma rose from 3,255 between 1981 and 1983 to 5,429 from 1993 to 1995. The report estimated that the number of Americans who suffer from chronic illness will climb from 90 million in 1999 to 150 million by 2030.

Haven't we all either experienced or witnessed chronic conditions such as arthritis, diabetes, or heart disease that have a negative effect on the quality of life of a loved one? We continue to suffer as ability to function declines and the will to persevere gives way to passive attempts towards improving our own health. The CDC estimates that arthritis and other rheumatic conditions that currently affect one in every six people (43 million) will continue to escalate to more than 60 million Americans by 2020. This is the leading cause of disability in the United States and is estimated to cost almost $65 billion annually in medical care and lost productivity.

As chronic illnesses continue to overburden our health-care system, our society and its medical providers strive to find successful options for turning the tide of chronic debilitating disease in our country.

The Homeopathic Option: Purpose of the Pellets

The sixteenth-century philosopher and physician, Paracelsus, is quoted as saying, "Those who merely study and treat the effects of disease are like those who imagine that they can drive away the winter by brushing the snow from the door. It is not the snow that causes winter, but the winter that causes the snow." This illustrates one of the basic therapeutic principles in homeopathy that recognizes that all symptoms of illness are merely expressions of imbalance and disharmony within the whole person, and that it is the patient who needs treatment, not the disease.

Samuel Hahnemann, a German physician, chemist, linguist, and historian of medicine, discovered a different systematic approach to medicine in the late 1700s that would become homeopathy. He was dissatisfied with the state of medical practice and thought that the methods he was taught did more harm than good. In *Organon of the Medical Art* (O'Reilly, 1996), he writes about the current state of medical treatments. "This is a very faulty, much symptomatic treatment wherein only a single symptom, thus only a small part of the whole, is one-sidedly provided for." He continues to describe the quick but temporary treatment of persistent diseases during his era. "Frequently reoccurring pains of all sorts were suppressed for a short time with feeling-benumbing opium, then they always came back heightened, often intolerably heightened or other far-worse maladies came in their place."

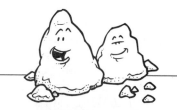

Natural Nuggets

Homeopaths have observed for the past two centuries that unless the entire person is healed, the symptoms that are driven away by medications will reoccur as the same or similar condition. You may also witness a decline of health as symptoms are suppressed by ongoing medications.

Engineering Your Migraine

Hindsight is truly 20/20. This explains why one way homeopaths learn about the therapeutic actions of the homeopathic remedies is through successfully treated patients' stories, or cured cases as they are commonly referred to. The end result usually follows the basic tenets of good homeopathic practice in that the patient has regained good overall physical, mental, and emotional health and the condition he came in with is gone and he is no longer dependent on any homeopathic remedies, conventional medications, or therapy. Here is a case from my own practice.

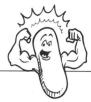

Potent Pellets

Organon of the Medical Art, written by Dr. Samuel Hahnemann, was first published in 1810. The sixth and final edition was completed in 1842, the year before he died. The book was for the general public, not just medical professionals. His work documents the evolution of his thoughts on the nature of disease and healing. My favorite translation is by Wenda Brewster O'Reilly (1996).

Frank is Mr. Project. Whether he was at home or at work, he was always busy with something. He was an engineer by profession who had an important managerial position of implementing the company-wide software transition. At home, he would relax by building an addition onto his home and remodeling several other rooms. He came to see me for the treatment of debilitating migraine headaches that were so severe he would have to leave work or be confined to a dark room for several hours of the day until the headache lessened. He couldn't stand the downtime. He had deadlines to maintain. At the same time, he felt his boss was watching him carefully because of Frank's critical role in guiding the company through the new software. With so much going on, he said, "I'm just trying to hold on." He was excellent at his job, disciplined, with a good eye for details, but migraines put him way behind schedule.

After listening to him for more than an hour and reviewing his complete system, I prescribed Cuprum Metallicum, the homeopathic form of copper, a common element.

After Frank took the homeopathic remedy over the next few months, the migraines he'd experienced since his teenage years disappeared. He was still busy at work, but without the sense that he was under so much pressure. He was less serious, laughed and smiled more often, and his family said he was easier to have fun with. As of this writing, he has not taken a dose of his remedy or any other medication for almost three years and has not experienced another migraine.

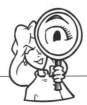

Curious Clues

Here are some hints for choosing Cuprum Metallicum (Scholten, 1996):

- ➤ Focus on task, work, duty
- ➤ Ability
- ➤ Maintaining
- ➤ Perfectionism
- ➤ Observed, criticism
- ➤ Order, routine
- ➤ Holding on
- ➤ Fear of failure

Many of the people who will most benefit from this remedy have a self-identity inseparable from their work or profession. They take on responsibility even when it's not their job. The illnesses usually occur during a period when they have to work too hard to force order and control while trying to maintain whatever they feel is normal. They can eventually be worn down by the effort and develop anxiety and fears at the prospect that their world is no longer in their control.

The Science Behind Homeopathy

Patients frequently ask me, "How does this stuff work?" There is a natural curiosity in a world where science has dominated for centuries. I encourage you to read on with a healthy skepticism and, if so inclined, obtain the studies mentioned and continue to learn how science is catching up to the potent pellets of homeopathy (see Appendix B, "Further Reading," for a complete list of all references cited in this book).

However, what and whose science do we count on for accurate and reliable information? Samuel Hahnemann based his medicine on observable or empirical studies of his patients, not the so-called science of the day that would later prove itself to be unsubstantiated fanciful theories without medical merit.

During the nineteenth century, physicians and scientists were in conflict over the causes of disease and the most appropriate way to treat it. It's no wonder that homeopathy came under heavy criticism despite its undeniable clinical effects. The basic sciences of biology, anatomy, chemistry, and physics were in their infancy. It is only recently that a growing body of scientific evidence has accumulated to begin explaining and even to prove the theories that homeopathy has witnessed in patients for the last 200 years.

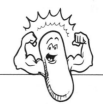

Potent Pellets

In 1833, disease was still thought of in many conventional medical circles as an imbalance between humors of the body: yellow and black bile, phlegm, and blood. The therapeutic agent of choice even during the era of "hospital medicine" in France was leeches for bloodletting. Forty million leeches were imported that year for bloodletting; the health of the average person went unchanged (Golub, 1994).

The Cluster Theory: Would You Like Ice in Your Water?

One of the challenging aspects of homeopathic theory has been that continual diluting and adding kinetic energy (the energy of motion) through shaking of medicines has a viable effect on the solution that is created. Dr. Shui-Yin Lo, senior research scientist with American Technologies Group of Los Angeles and visiting associate professor in chemistry at the California Institute of Technology, presented breakthrough research in 1997 at the Homeopathic Research Network meeting held in San Francisco.

Dr. Lo's research found that when a solution is diluted, placed in water, and shaken, as in homeopathic preparations, the water surrounding the solution begins to harden and form crystals or even ice at room temperature. He found the "IE clusters" (*I* for "ice" and *E* for "formed through electromagnetic forces rather than by temperature") of water measured by quantum electrodynamic calculations were not formed by simple dilution or shaking alone. Only the combination of these two actions, which are similar processes to the way homeopathic medicines are prepared, yielded the unique cluster formations. Dr. Lo went on to find that if the solution is further diluted and vigorously shaken, the concentration of the solid water clusters increases.

The "electromotive force" of water can be measured by putting two identical stainless steel electrodes in water and measuring the potential. Normal water shows no potential, while IE water shows an electromotive force.

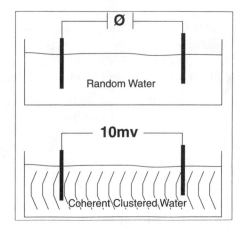

For the last two centuries, homeopaths have argued that each remedy has a unique action and effect on our body. Dr. Lo has been able to prove that the unique shape of the concentration is determined by the original substance that was put into chemical solution. This is one of the first studies that I am aware of that demonstrates the validity of many of the homeopathic principles that have governed its practice during the last 200 years.

The shape of the crystals is unique to the original substance.

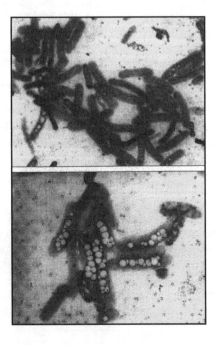

More research will certainly be coming from Dr. Lo, but if seeing is believing, then we've all got the first glimpses of what may prove many of the homeopathic theories of how a remedy can be diluted and still be active.

Homeopathic Human Studies: The Proof Is in the People

Homeopathic remedies are first tested on humans during a rigorous analysis called proving (see Chapter 6, "Where Do Homeopathic Remedies Come From?") The last two decades have seen an increased interest in homeopathic research due to its nontoxic, cost-effective potential. The *British Medical Journal 302* dated February 9, 1991, included a review of 25 years of clinical research on homeopathy. As Dana Ullman points out in *Homeopathic Medicine for Children and Infants* (Ullman, 1992), of the 107 controlled clinical trials, 81 showed successful results from homeopathic medicines, which suggests promising possibilities for treatment.

Homeopathic medicines treat a variety of complaints as shown by the collection of research outlined in Dr. Bill Gray's recent publication, *Homeopathy: Science or Myth?* Dr. Gray's review includes a study on acute pediatric diarrhea in Nicaragua by Jennifer Jacobs, M.D., M.P.H. The story was published in *Pediatrics* (1994) and shows dramatic reduction of symptoms well beyond random chance. The test protocols gave patients an individualized selected homeopathic remedy, and the results were qualified to meet conventional scientific standards.

I've given you a brief introduction to an expanding body of homeopathic research that will reassure the many individuals and families who rely on homeopathic care and satisfy even the most skeptical among us as to the potential benefits of homeopathy. I encourage you to continue your studies of homeopathy by picking up some of the books listed in Appendix B.

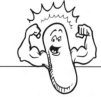

Potent Pellets

In 1997 the Homeopathic Medicine Research Group, established by Directorate Commission XII E of the European Union Commission, published a comprehensive report on a two-year study of homeopathic research. They concluded there was sufficient evidence of effectiveness to continue to develop more research into homeopathy.

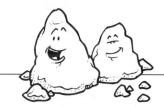

Natural Nuggets

Ninety women in their last month of pregnancy were given a combination remedy of five homeopathic medicines. The women given this mixture spent 40 percent less time in labor and had a 25 percent reduction in complications during birth as compared to the women given a placebo (Ullman, 1992).

The Least You Need to Know

➤ Because of the diluted solutions, homeopathic medicines are safe, nontoxic, and nonhabit forming.

➤ Homeopathic providers help to restore your whole health on a physical, mental, and emotional level.

➤ Your individual characteristics and symptoms assist your homeopath in selecting the most helpful remedy.

➤ Chronic diseases threaten to profoundly change the quality of our lives. Homeopathic care can be an important ally in attaining the best health possible.

➤ Recent discoveries enable scientific studies to support the theories and effectiveness of homeopathic medicines.

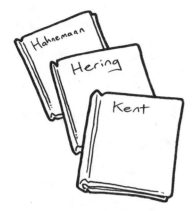

Chapter 2

The Evolution of Homeopathy

In This Chapter

➤ Learn how homeopathy was discovered

➤ Review the ups and downs of homeopathic medicine in the United States

➤ Look at the central controversies and objections to homeopathy

➤ Meet the key creators of homeopathy and understand their passion and purpose

---

The history of homeopathy reminds me of a roller coaster ride. The slow ascent carries the anticipation that something dynamic is about to happen. The view from the top is spectacular, and as you plunge downward you tell yourself that everything will be all right. Unexpected twists and turns, challenges met and surmounted, leave you feeling that you have not only survived but have overcome your fears and obstacles. Whew!

Get strapped in as you discover the beginning of homeopathy at a time when conventional medicine was struggling with finding solutions for disease. Ride along as I show you how, even at its infancy, homeopathy was able to effectively treat epidemics and gain rapid acceptance as a viable treatment option. Hold on through the dramatic increase in popularity of homeopathy through the training of medical professors, opening of schools, and its spread to the United States. Prepare to get slammed in a corkscrew upside-down loop as a head-to-head confrontation with conventional medicine occurs. Meet some of the medical practitioners who followed their deep beliefs, exercising patience and persistence during an often-tormenting ride.

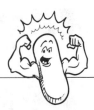

Potent Pellets

During the middle to late seventeenth century, amulets were thought to cure disease. A typical amulet, prepared at the proper phase of the moon and worn around the neck or wrist, might contain pulverized foods, specified quantities of first menstrual blood of a young maiden, white arsenic, pearls, corals, or Oriental emeralds. Today, receiving a pearl necklace or an emerald bracelet as a gift may also feel like a cure–all.

Dose of Info

Medicine comes from the Latin verb *medico*, which means "*to drug*," while **physician** comes from the Greek verb *phusis*, which means *nature*. Some view the practice of medicine in this country as increasingly revolving around chemical drug therapy and limiting the options of its doctors. Homeopaths utilize many substances from nature, as did the early Greek physicians.

As you exit the ride, you'll be exhilarated at how homeopathy has not only survived the medical political process but has emerged as one of the best hopes among complementary medical procedures for the safe, effective, and inexpensive treatment of our mounting health concerns.

Homeopathy Is Born Among Amulets and Leeches

If you were to get sick during the late 1600s or 1700s, what would be your options? There was no television for advertisers to educate you on their products and no Internet to surf through hours of expert advice. If you lived in Europe or England, your choices depended on whether you lived in the city or the country and how affluent you were. If you had money, a university-educated man with gentlemanly bearing would come to your home or bedside, give you a diagnosis and advice, and stop by regularly to see how you were doing.

According to Edward S. Golub, Ph.D., author of *The Limits of Medicine,* the physicians trained in *medicine* at that time "studied natural philosophy because the purpose of the *physician* was to preserve health and prolong life; healing was only a small part of what they did. Physician's education involved little if any clinical training. When they received this doctor-of-medicine training, it signified that they were learned men who knew a great deal of natural philosophy and moral philosophy" (Golub, 1994).

At that time, your doctor could identify your condition and support you as it ran its course. You would also be given philosophical and moral advice. He may have tried to help with different treatments to rid you of evil humors by purging you through vomiting, diarrhea, sweating, or blood letting with our old friends, the leeches. These treatments were often harsh and weakened the patient significantly, but since medicine had not changed significantly over the last 200 years, the patients' and doctors' expectations were the same.

People were still getting sick and looking for answers. Excluding the wealthy, most people in England at this time sought medical care from people supplementing their income through medicine. Your local grocery store would carry drugs; blacksmiths would pull teeth and set bones; medical charlatans and *quacks* traveled the countryside dispensing elixirs to the waiting sick and suffering.

With medicine holding onto the old-school concepts of evil humors, religiosity, and resisting the new philosophy of the new sciences such as biology and anatomy that had just begun to be discussed, the general public was still suffering and something had to be done.

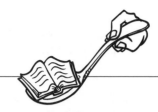

Dose of Info

According to *A Dictionary of Word Origins* by John Ayto, **quack** is derived from an old English word *quack-salver*, someone who quacks or boasts about the healing powers of their salves or medicines. Doctors at this time were gentlemen who would never lower themselves to boasting.

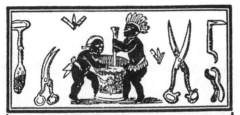

Good News to the Sick.

Veragainſt *Ludgate* Church, within *Black-Fryers* Gate-way, at *Lillies-Head*, Liveth your old Friend Dr. *Caſe*, who faithfully Cures the Grand P—, with all its Symptoms, very Cheap, Private, and without the leaſt Hindrance of Buſineſs. *Note*, He hath been a Phyſitian 33 Years, and gives Advice in any Diſtemper *gratis*.

All ye that are of *Venus* Race,
Apply your ſelves to Dr. *Caſe*;
Who, with a Box or two of PILLS,
Will ſoon remove your painſull ILLS.

Dr. Case was writing and practicing medicine in London, England, during the late seventeenth and early eighteenth centuries. This handbill is typical of his wit and quackery. Another handbill read, "Dear Friends, let your disease be what God will, pray to him for a cure. Try Case's skill."

(Source: Quacks of Old London, *C. J. Thompson)*

Thinking Outside the Box

Samuel Hahnemann (1755–1843) was a young student and doctor in Germany during the medical turmoil of the time. Several philosophies and authorities about disease rapidly came and went or coexisted, confusing the general public and their physicians. Samuel Hahnemann was a brilliant student whose dedication to understanding led him to become a physician, a chemist, a linguist, and a medical historian. Disillusioned with medicine, he believed that the methods taught in school did more harm than good. He quit the practice of medicine and began translating medical texts. While he was translating the Scottish physician William Cullen's book of *Materia Medica* in 1790, he took particular notice of the *toxicology* of Peruvian bark.

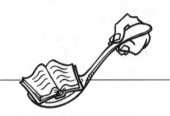

Dose of Info

According to *Webster's New World Dictionary* and *A Dictionary of Word Origins*, **toxicology** is the science of poisons, their effects, and their antidotes. The underlying word *toxic* is derived from a Latin word *toxicum*, which has roots in the Greek word *toxon* or bow. The first use of a toxin originally meant the poison that is put on arrows to shoot from a bow.

Peruvian bark, or Cinchona, from which the drug quinine is derived, is used to treat malaria. Hahnemann noted that the toxic effects of the bark produced the same symptoms of the disease it was known to cure. He began to experiment on himself to understand how this occurred. He began to form ideas from his experiments and hypothesized that the bark produced an *artificial disease* when given to a healthy person, which would then stimulate the body to overpower the natural illness of a sick person.

In 1796, Hahnemann published his first work on homeopathy, titled *Essay on a New Principle or Ascertaining the Curative Powers of Drugs with a Few Glances at Those Hitherto Employed*. He conducted studies on healthy individuals called provings (see Chapter 6, "Where Do Homeopathic Remedies Come From?") and felt that the body's natural abilities should be stimulated to effectively deal with disease. He based his theories on clinical observations instead of the humoric imaginations of the times. You'll learn more about Samuel Hahnemann later in this chapter.

Homeopathy Emerges in Mainstream Medicine

Samuel Hahnemann's new medical philosophy was originally greeted with the same skepticism that every new medicine of the month was given. However, there began to be an important difference between the conventional medicine of the times and Hahnenmann's philosophy that would distinguish homeopathy as a true healing art … it worked.

Samuel Hahnemann continued experimenting, teaching, and writing. Homeopathy soon gained credibility with its dramatic cure rate during epidemics of scarlet fever and cholera. These results caused his medical practice to swell as patients and even royalty traveled long distances from surrounding countries to consult with him. Homeopathy spread rapidly through Europe as a result of the successful treatments of the epidemics and chronic diseases of the time. It's no wonder that this safe, inexpensive, and effective therapy would catch on and continue to spread throughout India, South America, and the United States.

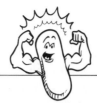

Potent Pellets

Homeopathy hits a home run in the United States:

➤ 1824—European M.D.s who were first- or second-generation students of Samuel Hahnemann begin to practice in America.

➤ 1835—First American homeopathic medical school established.

➤ 1842—The first national medical association is formed, The American Institute of Homeopathy.

➤ 1890—Homeopathy is widely used by the general public and an estimated 25 percent of all U.S. doctors are homeopathic M.D.s.

In nineteenth-century America, homeopathy was extremely popular, contributing to the importance of recognizing personal hygiene and lifestyle as indicators of health. However, it wasn't always easy dealing with the conventional medicine of the time. Clashes between the two existing theories of medicine continued as each felt the other's methods were questionable and easily disproved. Conflict also began to grow within the homeopathic community as to the purest form of practice. In 1880 homeopathic physicians who felt the profession was straying from the original principles of homeopathy split off from the American Institute of Homeopathy to form the International Hahnemannian Association.

With pressures mounting from inside and outside the profession, the newly developed sciences of pathology, bacteriology, and immunity changed the focus of conventional medicine from elevation of symptoms to the elimination of the causes of disease. Homeopathy became more isolated in the medical community as homeopaths could not use these new sciences to demonstrate the basis for homeopathy's successful treatment of disease. During the middle to late 1800s, the American Medical Association (AMA), which formed two

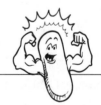

Potent Pellets

In 1911, the *Flexner Report on Medical Education* required medical educational standards to be based on conventional medical opinion. This resulted in the eventual elimination of homeopathic education at all medical schools by 1935.

years after the American Institute of Homeopathy, set policies in its organization and lobbied most medical associations to shun any professional or personal contact with homeopaths.

While homeopathy was flourishing in other parts of the world, it was slowly dying from the lack of quality education at U.S. medical schools. With the discovery of antibiotics and other technical advances in conventional medicine, fewer physicians were willing to face professional harassment and, as a result, homeopathy became even scarcer. Homeopathy was down, but not out.

The Criticism and Controversy

New ideas almost always come under fire of the established organizations. This was and still is the case with homeopathy. What follows is a sampling of the criticisms that are leveled at homeopathy.

➤ According to the National Council Against Health Fraud Inc. (NCAHF), a voluntary health agency that focuses on health misinformation, fraud, and quacks, the *Homeopathic Pharmacopoeia* has been included in the U.S. Food, Drug, and Cosmetics Act due to political influence and not scientific merit, giving the practice of homeopathy an unjustified legitimacy in medicine and the law.

➤ The NCAHF urges scientists to be proactive in opposing the marketing of homeopathic products because of their "conflicts with known physical laws." They continue to state in their position paper, titled *Guide to Coverage of Complementary and Alternative Medicine, 2000 Edition,* "that state and federal regulatory agencies are urged to take strong enforcement action against violators of standards in manufacturing, including disciplinary health professionals who practice homeopathy. States are urged to abolish homeopathic licensing boards."

➤ The report continues to scrutinize the dilution and potentizing of substances by saying that homeopaths have failed to prove its validity. Homeopathic practitioners are labeled "quacks and charlatans," with most of the public appeal generated from the homeopaths' personal attention and careful listening to the emotional state of the patient. The science and technology behind both of these concepts will be discussed fully in Chapter 5, "How to Make a Homeopathic Remedy."

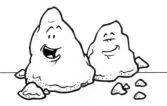

Natural Nuggets

Many of the criticisms against homeopathy state that good studies are not available. This comment continues despite the growing number of well-conducted research studies: "Sprained Ankle Pain," Zell et. al., 1988, and Thiel and Bohro, 1991: "Influenza," Ferley et. al., 1989; "Hay Fever," Reilly, 1986.

As homeopathic education continues to improve and new scientific research and theories reach those who have minds open enough to read them, perhaps these biased remarks will give way to more balanced and firm ways to ensure safety and effectiveness of homeopathic products and services.

The Pioneers: Take Less Young Man, Take Less!

Whenever there is new territory to explore, pioneers of every land or profession risk it all in the belief that they are doing the right thing. They often push past the comments of their peers to honor a core belief that has not been proven yet, but in which they have seen enough to know the path is worth pursuing. In homeopathy, there have been numerous practitioners from many countries who have greatly contributed to the successful treatment of patients while elevating the science and educational standards. I will introduce you briefly to three such pioneers, knowing that you will find many more when you continue your studies of this medical art.

Samuel Hahnemann Put the Homeo in Homeopathy

Born to a poor German family in 1755, Samuel Hahnemann early on developed a thirst for knowledge. He learned nine languages and read most medical books published during his time. Earning his degree as a medical doctor in 1791, he practiced conventional medicine for nine years until he became disillusioned by its effects.

While translating a medical book, he discovered by accident that Peruvian Chinchona bark, once ingested, gave him the same symptoms of malaria that the bark was used to treat. He performed diligent trials describing his new findings by coining a Latin phrase *similia similibus curantur*—"like is cured by like" and named the new therapy *homeo* (similar) *pathy* (suffering). He conducted many years of experiments verifying theories and continuing to dilute substances and giving minimal doses to reduce any side effects. He was ridiculed by his contemporaries despite the growing number of successful cases he treated including epidemics of scarlet fever and cholera. In 1810 Hahnemann published the first of six editions of *Organon of the Medical Art,* a book on his theories of the origins and treatment of disease.

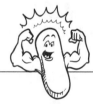

Potent Pellets

According to the Web site www.homeopathy.org, in 1821 cholera swept through Central Europe. This led to the first widespread use of homeopathy, which had a 96 percent cure rate as compared with conventional medicine's 41 percent cure rate.

Samuel Hahnemann (1755–1843) founded a new medical system he named homeopathy.

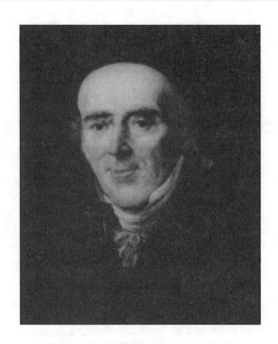

Constantine Hering—The Father of American Homeopathy

Constantine Hering got into homeopathy in an indirect manner. Born January 1, 1800, in Oschatz, Germany, he developed an interest in medicine and studied at Leipzig University. A professor asked him to write a paper to disprove Hahnemann's recently published book *Organon of Rational Medicine*. The project backfired, for after reading the book he wrote his doctoral thesis on *De Medicina Futura* (The Medicine of the Future). Hering practiced homeopathy as the physician-in-attendance for the governor of Surinam. He began to focus his attention on developing new homeopathic medicines and would send notes of his work to Hahnemann for his feedback.

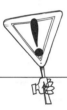

Caution Keeper

While trying to find an improved substitute for the cowpox inoculation, which Hering felt was dangerous, his enthusiasm led him to performing numerous self-tests of snake venoms, one of which left him paralyzed on his right side.

In 1833 he sailed for the United States, first settling in Martha's Vineyard, the site he and the crew were able to get to after their ship was destroyed in a storm. He moved to Philadelphia in 1848, where he opened the Hahnemann Medical College of Pennsylvania.

Hering and his students treated more than 50,000 patients a year and trained a total of 3,500 homeopaths. He organized his notes into *The Guiding Symptoms of Our Materia Medica* in 1879—the year before he died.

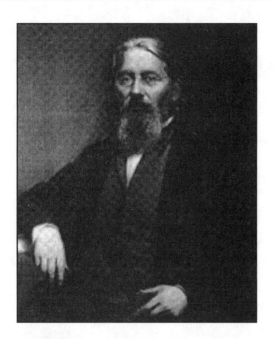

Constantine Hering (1800–1880)—the Father of American Homeopathy.

James Tyler Kent—The Organizer

Kent was a private man who practiced conventional medicine in St. Louis where he became interested in homeopathy following the successful treatment of his wife by Dr. Richard Phelan, a graduate from Hering's Hahnemann College. In 1888 he became a consulting physician at Philadelphia's new all-homeopathic hospital. It was there that he founded a legendary postgraduate school. His beliefs in treating a patient's mental, emotional, spiritual, and physical body simultaneously required new therapies and practices, which have evolved homeopathy into the medicine we have today.

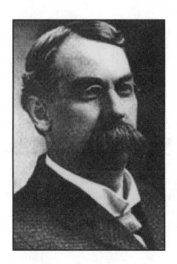

James Tyler Kent (1849–1916) further developed homeopathic insight and philosophy and developed a better-organized system of referencing symptoms with homeopathic medicines.

American Homeopathy Today: The Comeback Kid

Homeopathy declined in the United States from the 1940s to the late 1970s. A few practitioners carried on the traditions and created new innovations. The rise in popularity of homeopathy began with the search for better health from numerous therapies discussed in Chapter 1, "What Is Homeopathy and How Does It Work?" as complementary alternative medicine. The National Center for Homeopathy now runs the postgraduate courses that were taught by the American Foundation for Homeopathy in 1922.

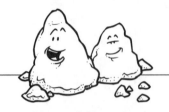

Natural Nuggets

Homeopathy can usually be practiced legally by those with degrees that entitle them to practice medicine, such as Doctors of Osteopathy or Naturopathy, dentists, acupuncturists, chiropractors, and veterinarians.

The National Center for Complementary Alternative Medicine (NCCAM) is receiving a record amount of federal funding to set up fair and balanced testing procedures for many therapies, including homeopathy. "The manufacture and sale of homeopathic medicines is regulated by the Food and Drug Administration (FDA). Homeopathic medicines are legal in this country and states regulate the practice of the estimated 3,000 practitioners of which 500 are M.D.s" (*The State of Healthcare in America*, 1998).

The use of homeopathic medicine under the laws of most states for self-care of acute conditions is available to everyone in the country, as seen by the availability of over-the-counter homeopathic products at many health food stores and retail outlets. High-quality homeopathic education for medical professionals and the general public is now available across America, ensuring that quality and accurate care continue to thrive as an option for you and your family.

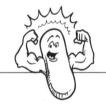

Potent Pellets

According to *Landmark Report* (1998), 61 percent of those surveyed in a national study said they were likely to use homeopathy as part of their health care.

Homeopathy was developed during an era of general confusion and turmoil in conventional medicine. There was a desperate search by many to learn the origins of disease and the most effective treatments. Samuel Hahnemann received abundant praise and criticism for his new medical art that had so much success with the epidemics that crippled European countries. Homeopathy quietly spread throughout many countries, but was met with overwhelming criticism in the United States.

At the turn of the twentieth century there were 22 homeopathic medical colleges in the United States and one out of five doctors used homeopathy. The growing acceptance and enthusiasm toward a mechanical/technical model of our bodies and disease pushed homeopathy further into the background as it struggled to prove its theories with the new sciences. By 1910 only 15 homeopathic colleges remained and, by the late 1940s, no courses were taught in the United States.

There has been a strong interest and rise in homeopathic education, research, and quality practice since the 1970s fueled by the general public, again searching for better health. The future looks bright for homeopathy with a more unified profession committed to high standards of education and continued emphasis on quality research and care so that this gentle medicine will always be available as an option for your health care.

The Least You Need to Know

➤ Homeopathy was discovered at a time when leeches, amulets, and harsh purgatives treated the ills of the world.

➤ Samuel Hahnemann, a German physician, discovered that medicines hold the key to their best use by studying their effects on healthy people.

➤ Homeopathy spread rapidly through many countries of the world, but was eventually met with great opposition in the United States.

➤ The first national medical association, The American Institute of Homeopathy, was founded in 1842. Two years later the American Medical Association (AMA) was formed.

➤ Continual clashes ensued between these groups almost eliminating homeopathy until the 1970s when homeopathy saw a resurgence.

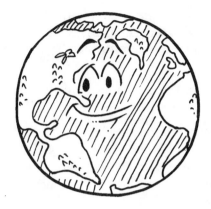

Chapter 3

Homeopathy Around the World

> ### In This Chapter
>
> ➤ Learn what happened when homeopathy went global
>
> ➤ Find out how homeopaths have organized and educated themselves
>
> ➤ Homeopathic hospitals? You bet!
>
> ➤ Discover how other countries have integrated homeopathic care into their health system

Perhaps you've seen enticing advertisements promising a tour of 10 countries in 5 days. This chapter won't cover as much territory as that; however, we will take a look at what other countries have done with the practice of homeopathy since its inception 200 years ago. We'll also visit organizations that serve as home base for many of the leading homeopaths in the world.

Homeopathic Organizations: Getting It Together

Professional organizations form to share valuable information between colleagues, discuss and implement standards of care and education, and affect legislation. Homeopathic organizations have grown to mirror the spread of this medical art. A large organization usually means that homeopathy is well entrenched in the culture and medical practices of the country.

The Club Close-Ups: Stand and Be Counted

The following information has been supplied by an extensive 10-country survey compiled by the European Council for Classical Homeopathy (ECCH). This organization is dedicated to keeping high standards and communication in the homeopathic community:

➤ India has the largest number of homeopaths. There are more than 125,000 registered practitioners.

➤ In France 18,000 homeopathic practitioners, 32 percent of all general practitioners, 700 veterinarians, and 2,000 dentists prescribe homeopathy.

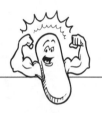

Potent Pellets

Homeopathy has enjoyed the patronage of royalty from the time that Samuel Hahnemann treated many of the royal houses of Germany. According to Paul Downey in *Homeopathy for the Primary Healthcare Team,* many of these nobles were relatives of Queen Victoria. A patron of Hahnemann's at one time was the father of Prince Albert, who later married Queen Victoria of England (Downey, 1997).

➤ The British association of professional homeopaths, The Society of Homeopaths, has 2,500 members.

➤ The Norwegian Homeopathic Association has about 400 full members and 150 student members.

➤ The Australian Institute of Homeopathy was formed in 1946 and later became the most popular national organization, The Australian Homeopathic Association, of which 80 percent of homeopathic practitioners are members.

➤ The New Zealand Homeopathic Society, founded in 1951 by a lay practitioner, Alfred G. Grove, has about 100 professional homeopaths as members.

Whether you're in the United States or traveling overseas, if you do not have the name of a recommended homeopath, the next best step is to contact the national organizations. These societies reflect the standards and training of the professionals in that region. As you will be reading, these standards can vary considerably from country to country.

Homeopathic Education Overseas

This section provides a closer look at the training involved in becoming a homeopathic practitioner in various countries.

The Education Station

In European countries, many medical doctors have done additional training in homeopathy and an increasing number of professional homeopaths who train solely in homeopathy as a clinical discipline treat patients for a wide range of conditions. The levels of education vary from country to country:

➤ In India, official recognition of education and training of homeopaths is equal to that of medical doctors. There are 125 officially recognized homeopathic schools where the education takes from 4.5 to 5.5 years full time.

➤ A homeopath approved in Norway has from three to five years of part-time education, depending on his medical background.

➤ Denmark has only one school of homeopathy, which offers a four-year part-time degree broken into 544 hours of homeopathy and 350 hours of general medicine.

➤ German homeopaths vary greatly. For doctors to earn the title "homeopath," they must have two years of clinical work, three years of theoretical work, or one year in a hospital in a department of homeopathy, plus six months of additional courses. About 10 percent of homeopaths are self-trained, while most attend private homeopathic school, full- or part-time.

➤ France offers two ways to get homeopathic education: private schools or universities. Some of the private schools are run by homeopathic manufacturers such as Boiron or Dolisos. Seven universities organize a one-year postgraduate course, while seven others offer a three-year training cycle. Four French schools of veterinary medicine provide structured training in homeopathy.

➤ In England there are no officially recognized national standards. Teaching and training varies from short courses of five weeks to three years full-time.

Potent Pellets

King George VI of England used homeopathy and even named one of his racehorses after a remedy. The horse, Hypericum, won the purse in 1949. Today members of the British royal family still use homeopathy (Downey, 1997).

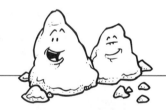

Natural Nuggets

What's in a name? If you're looking for a homeopath overseas, you'd better remember these titles: Germany—*Heilpuaktiker;* Norway—*Homeopath MNHL;* France—no official title; England—*RS Hom* or *UKHMA;* India—*homeopath.*

Homeopathic Association of Switzerland.

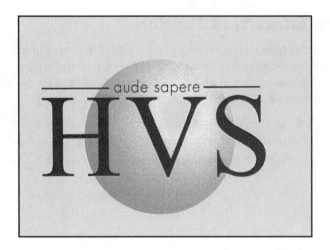

As you can see, the training varies among countries as to the educational requirements of a homeopath. Careful questioning about the practitioner's training and skill will most often yield the best results for you and your family.

Homeopathic Hospitals: A Dose of Caring

Four out of the ten countries surveyed by the European Council for Classical Homeopathy still operate homeopathic hospitals or hospitals with homeopathic wards. In these medical centers, you are treated with the best possible care, which may include a homeopathic option:

Dose of Info

The word **hospital** comes from the Latin word *hospes,* which means *guest* or *host,* and the hospital as we know it comes from early Christian hospitals where acts of mercy could be carried out to a wide variety of those in need (Golub, 1994).

➤ In India, a total of 273 hospitals offer homeopathic treatment, 15 out of 20 municipal hospitals have homeopathic wards, and there are 8,865 homeopathic clinics for the poor.

➤ Many *hospitals* in Germany offer homeopathic medicines. Most of these are private institutions, and a fewer number offer classical homeopathy based on the whole person.

➤ The United Kingdom hosts five homeopathic hospitals. Of these, the hospital in Glasgow opened its first homeopathic dispensary in 1880. Approximately 15 percent of Scottish general practitioners have training in homeopathy.

Homeopathic treatments were available in some Australian hospitals up to the middle of this century. If you look carefully around at institutions in your area, you may find signs of the past prevalence of homeopathy. In my area, there's Hahnemann Hospital in Boston, which bears the name of homeopathy's founder, Samuel Hahnemann. Yet when I asked several practitioners who Hahnemann was, they did not know. Perhaps the future will see a greater integration of homeopathic and conventional medicine, inspired by the examples in the next section.

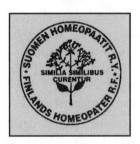

Homeopathic Association of Finland.

Homeopathy—Who Pays?

Homeopathy has been integrated into the health-care systems of several cultures, in both medical procedures and financial reimbursement. Take a look at the examples shown in this section. There are several models that may inspire you to push for your doctor working more closely with your homeopath for a more effective treatment. Examine how other countries pay for homeopathic treatment. Would you like your insurance company to cover this valuable service? It's time to write that letter, but first see how others are uniting the best of both worlds.

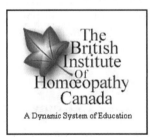

The British Institute of Homeopathy in Canada.

Integration Realization

Here are some examples of the way homeopathy, conventional medicine, and the accountants can get along in a health-care environment:

> ➤ Homeopathy has been integrated into the national health-care system in the United Kingdom for more than 50 years. Expenses for both consultations and medicines can be reimbursed when they are treated in a homeopathic hospital or referred to a homeopath by their medical doctor.

➤ Norwegian insurance companies may reimburse homeopathic treatment if there is a referral from a medical doctor.

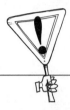

Caution Keeper

There is a great deal of variation from country to country between homeopathic providers and the way they charge for their services. Always make sure they are a match for your medical needs and your budget. When in doubt, call a state or national organization for guidance.

➤ Homeopathy is a benefit included in the national health-care system of Germany called the "besondere Therapierichtungen."

➤ Total French expenditures for homeopathy in 1994 were 1,366 million francs as compared to 2,380 million francs for other general practitioner care. Sixty-five percent of consultation and expenses for homeopathic medicines are eligible for reimbursement.

➤ The insurance companies in The Netherlands will refund homeopathic treatment provided the homeopath is a member of one of the national associations.

➤ There is no national health-care system in India, but government-subsidized homeopathic hospitals (273) and clinics (8,865) are available. Many conventional doctors are also trained in homeopathy, so there is a great deal of cooperation and referrals between practitioners.

Neither the European Commission nor the European Parliament have produced any positive statement on who may or may not practice homeopathy. The delivery of health-care services is considered to be a concern of each member state rather than one of the European Union.

The Least You Need to Know

➤ India has the largest number of homeopaths, with more than 125,000 registered practitioners.

➤ Homeopathic education varies, such as in Norway, which has a three- to five-year course of study depending on your medical background.

➤ The United Kingdom has five homeopathic hospitals, such as in Glasgow, which opened its doors in 1880.

➤ Sixty-five percent of consultations and homeopathic medicines are eligible for reimbursement in France.

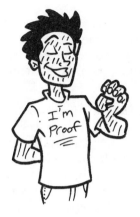

Chapter 4

Provings—The Proof Is in the Person

In This Chapter

➤ Poisoning versus proving

➤ Discover the hidden healing potential that is uncovered by a homeopathic proving

➤ Find out how examining the reactions of healthy people in a proving can benefit the sick

➤ Learn how many people can produce the same symptoms

➤ Take a peek at past provings

This chapter will untangle a unique feature of homeopathic medicine, "the proving of a remedy," and show you how it's all done, and why this information is amazingly accurate. You'll see what a proving reveals and how this extraordinary compilation of information yields rich details for our understanding of remedies.

What do you get when you put a group of provers into one room? A deep understanding of a homeopathic remedy that can only come from experiencing the effects first-hand. I'll share with you my own personal experiences of being a prover and the shocking similarities I shared with my colleagues during the process.

New homeopathic medicines are continually being proven. I'll tell you about one of the new and very familiar substances that could help our modern-day maladies.

What's Proved in a Proving?

How many times have you heard someone say, "Prove it"? It's a phrase we toss around most of the time as a jesting challenge. However, there's no joking around about the issues of illness and disease when it comes to accurately prescribing the best homeopathic remedies available.

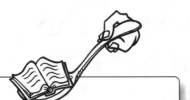

Dose of Info

A **homeopathic proving** is an artificial epidemic. All the individuals participating become a whole and unified organism. They share the same source and their vital forces merge. This is called the "as if one person" factor.

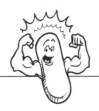

Potent Pellets

In a proving, healthy volunteers take a remedy with unknown properties (or placebo in a randomized fashion) and record any symptoms. The remedy then has subtle effects on the nervous system, immune system, digestive process, and so on. If described in great detail and with an eye to whatever is most peculiar and unique, a picture of the remedy gradually emerges.

Source: Gray, 2000

Homeopathic provings are the foundation of the accuracy of homeopathy. During this process (which will be discussed in more detail later in this chapter), a person takes a homeopathic medicine and records in great detail all of his or her thoughts and feelings—physical, emotional, and mental. The symptoms are filtered by excluding any feelings that the healthy person would have on his own and then combined with many others' experiences who have been taking the same substance at the same time. This forms a huge database that is used by practitioners to match the symptoms provers experience during their illness. The more detailed and accurate the proving notes are, the better possibility we as practitioners have of matching the symptoms of the prover and patient together.

Through diligent work, Dr. Hahnemann's skill and insights into homeopathic medicines increased through the process of provings. Once he found the process to be safe and had figured out the steps involved to do an accurate trial, he let his students and other doctors expand their knowledge of homeopathy through the process of proving a remedy. Women as well as men were involved because he theorized that disease would manifest in women differently than in men, a concept that has not always been part of all modern pharmaceutical testing.

Hahnemann found that diluted and succussed solutions (discussed in Chapter 5, "How to Make a Homeopathic Remedy") were more "potent" at producing a wide range of unique symptoms in an individual than the raw substance. This separated his provings from the toxicology or poisoning reports that were available on substances like lead and mercury, which had earlier been used in medicine. As people died, careful notes were taken of their symptoms. Using highly diluted substances, homeopaths are able to safely study many substances, even poisonous venoms, while acquiring a more complete understanding of all the areas where nonconventional medicine may help a sick person.

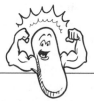

Potent Pellets

In *Organon of the Medical Art,* Samuel Hahnemann spells out basic requirements for being a prover. Could you be a prover? Here are the necessary characteristics:

➤ You are known to be credible and conscientious.

➤ You guard against mental and bodily exertion.

➤ You guard against all excesses and disturbing passions.

➤ You have no urgent business to deter one from proper observation, and, with good will, direct exact attention to oneself without being disturbed.

➤ You are bodily healthy (whatever *is* good health for you).

➤ You possess the necessary intellect to be able to name and describe one's sensibilities in distinct expressions.

Source: Paragraph 126, Organon of the Medical Art. *Wenda O'Reilly, 1996.*

Homeopathic medicines are proved using people who can describe every minute change in their bodies and minds, in contrast to other pharmaceuticals that are tested on animals or less rigorously reported by human test subjects. To date, more than 2,500 to 3,000 homeopathic medicines have been tested through provings.

The Proving of Chocolate— How Sweet It Isn't!

Chocolate, mmmmm! Just the name swishing from your mouth starts your mouth watering, as you remember the last succulent morsel you devoured. Jeremy Sher, a renowned Canadian

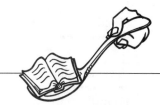

Dose of Info

Cocoa and **chocolate** are made from the edible seeds of the tropical American tree *Theobroma cacao.* The name *Theobroma* means food of the gods, while *cacao* is derived from the Aztec name for the cacao tree (Sher, 1994).

homeopath, chose chocolate to prove as a homeopathic medicine, because the substance is so pervasive in our society.

His first step was to find the "plain best quality of Belgian dark *chocolate* (unbranded)." Following the guidelines in the footnotes of paragraph 270 of the 6th edition of *The Organon,* (this sample) was triturated (rubbed, crushed, or ground into fine particles or powders) with lactose. The powder was then dissolved in water and alcohol and succussed 45 times to give it a homeopathic strength of 4c (see Chapter 5 or Appendix C, "Homeopathic Pharmacy Terminology"). "Potentization continued in liquid form using separate vials, 45 succussing and 90 percent alcohol as a dilutent at each step as per Hahnemann's instructions up to 200c." (Preparation of remedies will be further explained in Chapter 5.) The proving on chocolate was conducted with a careful grouping of symptoms recorded. A person who may benefit from the homeopathic form of chocolate would display symptoms similar to the ones listed in the following table.

A Sprinkle of Chocolate Symptoms

Mental
Affectionate or angry in the evening
Anger over small things
Unsympathetic or aversion for loved ones
Desire for darkness
Delusion of being alone in the world
Dreams of childbirth, darkness, death of relatives
Irritability, shouting, slamming doors

Nose
Coldness of tip of nose, stuffed up in a warm room

Sleep
Sleepless during menses

Hand
Dull pain in back of hand extending to the top, pressing pain in the forehead

Food
Aversion to butter, cooked foods, fats, and rich foods, ice cream
Desire for fruit juice, carbonated drinks, ice, chocolate, cold drinks, sweets, cayenne pepper

A Homeopathic Case for Chocolate

Sammy appeared to be a bright and engaging three-year-old boy brought in by his mother for behavior issues. During the course of our interview, I noticed that Sammy would nuzzle with his mom, then appeared to suddenly jerk away from her in anger and go off by himself while ignoring both of us. She said this was typical behavior. Often he would sit by himself in a darkened room, later complaining to her that he was all alone. Sometimes he would take her affection, while other times he would storm off in a huff, slamming his door behind him. At mealtime he was hard to please, with a strange list of foods he wanted like spicy foods, sodas, and sweets, and anything raw. Once you cooked his food, he would refuse it.

She was unable to change his mind and was very concerned that he would not outgrow this phase as her doctor had predicted. I gave him a homeopathic form of chocolate, and over the next six to eight weeks, his behavior and mealtime madness changed dramatically to more consistency at the dinner table and in his mother's arms.

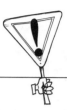

Caution Keeper

The World Health Organization (WHO) estimates that 25,000 deaths per year are due to pesticide usage in developing countries. Workers on cocoa plantations often slave in a cloud of chemical dust. In Brazil, powerful pesticides are sprayed on the cocoa crops, many of which have been banned in other countries (Sher, 1999).

The Homeopathic Proving of Carbon Dioxide (CO_2)

I was in a homeopathic course taught by Louis Klein, a well-respected practitioner from Vancouver, Canada, when he asked if we would like to participate in a large proving of a homeopathic substance, CO_2. We had all studied homeopathy for years, but most of us had never been involved in a proving. We had to decide whether this was a good time in our lives to devote the necessary amount of energy and concentration on this project, and if we were in good health ourselves.

I decided to go for it. This was a great opportunity to deepen my understanding of a remedy and the homeopathic process. I could choose either to be part of the administrative team, which collects and sorts the mounds of information we collected, or to be a prover and experience the essence of the remedy firsthand. Anyone who knows me can figure out I'm up for the adventure—I chose to be a prover.

I met with my *supervisor* who would do a two-hour interview with me to understand every aspect of my physical, mental, and emotional self. My supervisor and I discussed how we would communicate with each other several times a day to record all that would occur during the proving process, which lasted about a month.

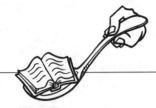

Dose of Info

Supervisors are experienced homeopaths who work with their proving partner to record every aspect of reported symptoms several times per day. They have a very thorough initial interview with their prover to be able to compare symptoms from before and after the proving.

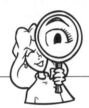

Curious Clues

Here are a few clues that would point you to the homeopathic remedy chocolate: alternating between affection and anger; retreating into darkness; having a strange feeling you are alone in the world; anger and irritability; desire for sweets, spicy foods, and aversion to cooked foods.

The Proving Process

I was given a small vial of white pellets and instructed to take them once a day for a few days, until I began to feel "something" that was different or unusual from my normal experiences. I didn't know whether I had a real remedy or a placebo. None of us except the master prover (Lou Klein) ever knew the identity of the remedy being proved.

I had a journal where I wrote detailed notes on my experiences at least twice a day, which I relayed to my supervisor who met with me or phoned one to two times a day. I reported all my experiences such as dreams of business, receiving gifts, or my waking experiences such as decreased appetite, a red blemish on my nose, and jaw pain. Each day I recorded the time I took a dose of the proving remedy. My concentration was focused although sometimes I experienced unusual confusion and mental fatigue. I experienced vivid dreams ranging in themes from feelings of being left behind to being abandoned and betrayed.

The feelings were strong and physical sensations such as a sharp stabbing sensation in the legs or headaches would come and go. I found myself experiencing life in a very difficult manner. I'm usually pretty centered, and I wasn't during this time. I wrote down and reported the emotions that resulted.

The Stages of a Proving

In his book *The Dynamics and Methodology of Homeopathic Provings*, Jeremy Sher describes these stages of a proving:

Stage one: Preparation—obtain proving supervisors, obtain potentized remedy, set up committees.

Stage two: Proving—prover takes remedy and reports to supervisor who notifies master prover.

Stage three: Extraction—the group meets to share information, first in small groups and then in larger groups. Finally the remedy is revealed.

Stage four: Collation—collected information is entered into a computerized database, symptoms are sorted.

Stage five: Repertorization—symptoms are organized in homeopathic form to be used by practitioners.

The Final Report: Circle the Wagons

All the provers, supervisors, committees, and coordinators met when the proving period was over. We shared our experiences in small groups and I was amazed at how many of my deep and intimate thoughts and feelings were also experienced with the same degree of intensity by other provers. Even dreams that I considered extremely personal were recounted by others who shared the same dream or else the feelings or themes that the dreams produced. When we finally got into a larger group and discussed the particulars of the provings, the same phenomenon occurred, except it was with a room full of people. This had been the experience of homeopaths over the last 200 years, but it was the first time I experienced something this curious and insightful.

What Do We Gain from Provings?

On a personal level, I gained an understanding of myself through the process of a thorough exam, continuous journaling, and reporting with a conscientious eye toward self-introspection. For a while, I embodied the remedy and will always remember that remedy and appreciate the inner nature of a remedy. Instead of just reading about a remedy in our materia medicas (books of homeopathic remedies and their proving symptoms) I walked away with a deeper understanding of the person who could benefit from this particular medicine. As a health-care provider, it helped to increase my sense of compassion for what my patients experience.

By observing myself, I became a better observer. I took only the amount of remedy that was needed to exhibit symptoms. The process was safe and when I stopped the proving, I felt great, in fact better than I had before! Hahnemann points out, "Let him not imagine that such small illnesses from taking proving medicines are generally detrimental to his health. On the contrary, experience teaches that, through the various attacks on a health condition, the prover's organism only becomes the more practiced in warding off everything from the external world. His health becomes more robust, as all experience teaches" (O'Reilly, 1996).

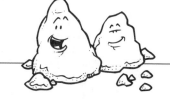

Natural Nuggets

A prover who is "sensitive," meaning his or her experiences are extreme, is of great usefulness to the proving. Any idiosyncrasies and unique sensations will bring a richer, more in-depth field of symptoms. A sensitive prover can make a great difference to the quality of the proving.

There will always be a need for qualified and accurate provings to explore new substances that may yield needed homeopathic medicines to help the suffering of others. As you have seen, the process involves a great commitment of time and employs meticulous information gathering that has been refined over the last 200 years of practice. A proving not only improves the practitioner's inner sense of a remedy, but improves the individual's overall health.

Next we'll take a look at how homeopathic remedies are made, their standards, and the key concepts of dilution and succussion.

The Least You Need to Know

➤ Homeopathic provers take an unknown substance until they produce symptoms that are meticulously recorded and collated to form a database of symptoms.

➤ Provers must be in good health, guard against all excesses during the process, and be conscientious at describing all feelings, physical, mental, or emotional.

➤ Homeopathic medicines are only tested on healthy humans, while other pharmaceuticals are animal tested.

➤ More than 2,500 to 3,000 homeopathic remedies have been proven.

➤ Provers gain insight into the real nature of remedies, increase their observational skills, and get a boost of good health.

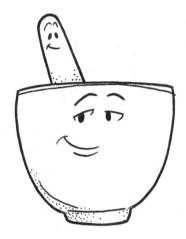

Chapter 5

How to Make a Homeopathic Remedy

In This Chapter

➤ Discover how homeopathic medicines are made from start to finish

➤ Learn how to potentize a remedy

➤ Is homeopathy safe? Examine the standards and the stats

➤ Learn how to read the labels

Homeopathy began its potentized practices before the Industrial Revolution that changed the way many things were made. In this chapter, you'll learn the time-honored procedures of making homeopathic medicines and find out how today's pharmacies have had to be ingenious to meet consumer demand for quality products. I'll be your tour guide through a pharmacy and show you the latest techniques and tips of the trade. What forms do homeopathic medicines come in? You'll learn about the power of the pellets and the liveliness of the liquids.

Homeopathic medicines are manufactured in accordance with the processes described in the *Homeopathic Pharmacopoeia of the United States,* which is the official manufacturing manual recognized by the FDA. Find out what this means for the safety of you and your family.

Have you ever been confused by looking at a vial of homeopathics? Not to worry. You'll be learning how to read the label along with a few insider tips on what the label really tells you. Keep turning the pages, as your familiarity with pharmacies begins.

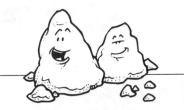

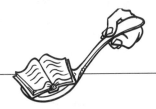

Dose of Info

Potentizing, a term coined by Dr. Samuel Hahnemann in the early 1800s, combines several serial dilutions of an original substance with vigorous shaking, known as succussion. The more a homeopathic remedy is diluted and shaken, the greater its healing strength or potential becomes.

The Making of a Remedy ... Succussion Discussion

I am frequently asked by patients, "How do they make a remedy?" While I'm happy to answer this question, I wonder how often they ask their conventional physician about the chemical drugs they are prescribed. My point is public perception. Although both homeopathic and chemical-based conventional medicines are regulated by the same agency, the FDA, public concern for homeopathics are higher due to their unfamiliarity. The manufacturing of homeopathics is strictly regulated, as you will learn. For now, let's make a remedy.

Dr. Samuel Hahnemann prepared the first homeopathic medicines in 1801. He found through his experiments that the process he called "potentizing," which involves continuous dilution or watering down of a substance, combined with vigorous shaking, helped solve two initial challenges:

1. The first was how to examine the properties and potential medical benefits of substances that are known to be poisonous, whether they are plants, minerals, or animal venoms.

2. The second was how to extract the greatest number of accurate and clear symptoms from the proving process so that the homeopath could effectively prescribe the remedies to match the symptoms of the sick. Hahnemann and the homeopaths that followed him found that *potentizing* remedies was the solution.

The continuous dilution of a substance not only reduces toxicity so that any substance can now be proved, but also increases the healing properties of a homeopathic medicine. Hahnemann found this out by experimentation; practitioners over the years have echoed his findings. Scientific research has recently confirmed that a diluted and shaken or succussed solution is more electromagnetically active than the original solution (see Chapter 1, "What Is Homeopathy and How Does It Work?"). This has been the stumbling block in logic for all homeopaths and their patients at one time or another.

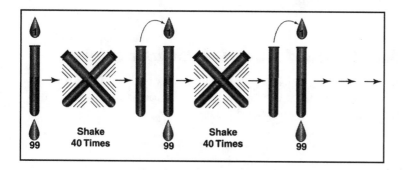

The process of "potentization": One drop of original substance is diluted in 99 drops of water. The vial is shaken (succussed) 40 times. Then 1 drop of that solution is diluted in another 99 drops of water, the resulting solution is shaken, and the process continues.

The Process to Potentize and Package

Now that you've seen how important the potentizing process is in theory, let's take a look at the whole process as we make a homeopathic remedy. It's worth mentioning again that the manufacturers of homeopathic medicines follow the standards established by the *Homeopathic Pharmacopoeia of the United States* (*HPUS*) and the regulatory requirements of the FDA.

The Process of Making a Homeopathic Medicine

1. Select pure raw material.
2. Grind (triturate) raw materials, if insolvable in water or alcohol, into a fine powder.
3. Preparation of liquid potencies by dilution and succussion.
4. Medicate blank pellets with liquid potencies.
5. Drying of medicated pellets.
6. Packaging of medicated pellets in vials.

The first step in making a remedy is to select the purest raw materials, preferably the same substance from the same area the medicine was originally proved from. Homeopathic manufacturers must be careful to choose only the best chemical and pollution-free source of materials. The materials are shipped to the manufacturing facility, which in most cases is a state-of-the art lab, where cleanliness is extremely important.

We'll be looking at Hahnemann Labs in San Rafael, California, for our tour of a homeopathic pharmacy. The staff looks prepped for surgery, complete with lab coats, hairnets, and shoe coverings. They are kept quite busy meeting and exceeding the strict manufacturing guidelines outlined by the FDA. All homeopathic processes are witnessed and recorded by at least two individuals, and meticulous records are kept of every substance from the time it enters their doors, as it's going through the homeopathic process, to the exacting labeling, packaging, and delivery of the homeopathic medicine.

Preparation of Soluble and Insoluble Substances

According to Hahnemann Labs, the materials that cannot be dissolved in water or alcohol (insoluble) need to be ground up or triturated. This process may take many hours; traditionally it was done by a mortar and pestle.

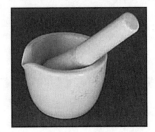

The mortar (bowl) and pestle (rod) were traditionally used to grind up substances that did not dissolve in water or alcohol. This process took many hours of strength and patience.

Now Hahnemann Labs does this work with a mechanical device called a ball mill. This is a design similar to a rock polisher or tumbler. Materials are placed in a jar along with 99 times as much lactose as the original substance. Very hard cylinders are also put into the jar which is placed on horizontal rollers. The rollers and cylinders continuously crunch the contents for hours until it becomes a fine powder that can be used to prepare liquid potencies.

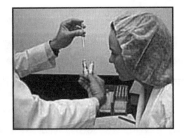

The first dilution of a substance makes the transformation from raw material (herb, mineral, and so on) to homeopathic medicine. Strict standards are applied to ensure quality homeopathic products.

Potentizing: Succuss or Bust

Substances that will dissolve in water or materials that are now powders are ready to prep for liquid potencies. This process is highly regulated, as it's the beginning of taking an herb or mineral and transforming it into a homeopathic medicine. First a dilution of one part original material to 99 parts liquid to create a $^1/_{100}$ ratio is made, and then this mixture is *succussed*.

At Hahnemann Labs, whenever a substance goes through this process, it must be witnessed by another person to make sure each critical step has been done correctly. The first 15 potencies are always prepared in separate vials, which is the Hahnemannian method.

Originally homeopaths succussed dilutions by slamming the vials against a book. This could take a while, and tire you out. At Hahnemann Labs, Michael Quinn, its founder, invented the Quinn potentizers, which are mechanical devices that ensure that successions are performed with the same number of strokes and with the same force on each stroke. The engineers who built the equipment even measured Michael Quinn's arm from elbow to closed hand to build a mechanical arm similar to the action of the founding homeopath's time-honored techniques.

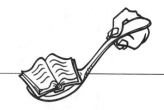

Dose of Info

According to Hahnemann Labs, **succussion** is the forceful pounding of the liquid dilution against a firm but resilient surface. Originally, homeopaths copied Samuel Hahnemann who used to succuss remedies by slamming them onto the surface of a book.

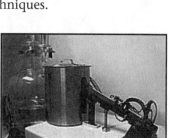

The Quinn potentizer at Hahnemann Labs mechanically re-creates the succussion of a dilution. The force of the succussion is equivalent to dropping—by gravity alone without any muscular action—your closed fist against a table from a height of 15 inches.

(Source: Hahnemann Labs)

The Final Process: Drip-Drying Away

We're so close to a homeopathic remedy, can you stand it? Each step has been carefully planned and documented. Cross-contamination has been avoided by rooms supplied with HEPA-filtered air and vents that constantly suck out air and vent it outside the building. The rooms are specialized so that no two processes take place in the same space.

Right now, I'm taking you to the medicating room. Small lactose pellets become homeopathic medicines by adding the newly potentized solution we've been following to a container of pellets. The container is shaken to distribute the solution evenly on the pellets and is allowed to penetrate the pellets for a minimum of five minutes. This step is also observed by witnesses and documented by triplicate paperwork. The pellets are dried by placing them on a clean white paper filter in a drying chamber that is also industrially vented so that air continuously flows across the pellets and to the outside. Dried pellets are packaged in several sizes, again in a room where air flow is designed to pull clean air over the pellets ensuring clean and safe packaging.

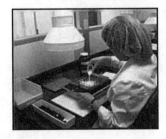

Dried pellets are packaged in well-ventilated rooms designed to ensure cleanliness and accuracy of packaging.

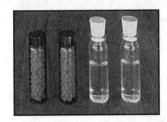

Homeopathic remedies are packaged in several sizes and potencies (strengths). Often they are stored in brown glass or plastic to lessen the possibility of damage by heat or light.

Manufacturing Standards: The Secret to Safety

High standards are what we expect when we buy a product, especially medicine. As all medicinal standards have evolved, so have the guidelines for the production of homeopathic products. When I give a homeopathic medicine to a patient, there is always a brief moment when his trust is tested by the fear of taking an unknown substance made by an unknown process. The general perception is that these could be made in someone's basement.

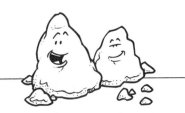

Natural Nuggets

Homeopathic medicines can be destroyed by excessive heat. During shipping, they may be vulnerable to the elements. Hahnemann Labs encloses a temperature gauge that turns black if the temperature in the package exceeds 120°F.

You now know how meticulously homeopathics are made, but you may be unaware of the standards they follow. The Federal Food, Drug, and Cosmetic Act adopted by Congress in 1938 gives the FDA the right to regulate drugs in the United States. Drugs are defined as those substances appearing in the official *United States Pharmacopoeia*, official *National Formulary*, or the official *Homeopathic Pharmacopoeia of the United States*. Homeopathic substances are recognized as official drugs by federal and most state governments.

The *Homeopathic Pharmacopoeia of the United States* is a compendium of substances used by homeo-pathic practitioners. It was originally published by the Pharmacopoeia Committee of the American Institute of Homeopathy in 1887. The committee, now called the Homeopathic Pharmacopoeia Revision Service (HPRS), currently meets three to six times per year to review new homeopathic remedies for inclusion into the official pharma-copoeia. This group is also responsible for setting guidelines for manufacturing and labeling of homeopathic remedies.

How to Read a Label

From 1938 through 1988 the FDA viewed all homeopathic medications as requiring a written prescription, according to Dr. Robert Middleton, clinical pharmacist at Alta Bates Medical Center in Berkeley, California. "During this time, the homeopathic industry was viewed by the FDA as very small and affecting a small segment of the population. Beginning in the 1970s, interest in homeopathy grew and an increasing number of homeopathic companies, both foreign and domestic began selling their products di-rectly to the public in health food stores, pharmacies, and through the mail." In 1988 new guidelines for the over-the-counter (OTC) sale of homeopathic products were set by the FDA's Compliance Policy Guide (CPG) and phased in over two years.

Here are some guidelines for over-the-counter homeopathic products:

➤ The remedy is used for self-limiting condi-tions that will resolve naturally over time.

➤ The remedy is indicated for use not requiring a medical diagnosis or monitoring.

➤ The contents of the entire package are not toxic.

Any remedy not meeting these conditions requires a prescription by a homeopathic practitioner.

As you have seen, homeopathic medicines are care-fully regulated and painstakingly prepared to com-ply with not only federal and state regulations, but with the homeopathic communities' demand for quality products. Regulatory agencies still rely heavily on the homeopathic community to have the knowledge and motivation to regulate this

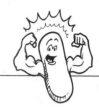

Potent Pellets

The Federal Food, Drug, and Cosmetic Act of 1938 was prima-rily authored by Dr. Royal B. Copeland, a homeopathic physi-cian who saw the value in homeo-pathic practices continuing in the United States.

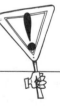

Caution Keeper

Drugs containing "official" homeopathic ingredients in combination with nonhomeo-pathic active ingredients are not considered homeopathic drugs. Manufacturers must provide clear labeling to avoid misleading the public.

growing industry. Only by adhering to these standards and guidelines can we be sure our patients and families are being given the high-quality homeopathic products they expect to use.

In the next chapter, we will look at specific families of remedies and the conditions they are uniquely suited to treat.

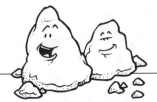

Natural Nuggets

Official guidelines for over-the-counter (OTC) homeopathics include (R. Middleton, 1993):

➤ The name of the medicine may be in Latin as well as English.

➤ Must list at least one major OTC indication for use.

➤ All prescription remedies must be accompanied by a package insert.

➤ Homeopathic remedies are exempt from expiration dating requirements.

The Least You Need to Know

➤ Potentizing a substance combines a series of dilutions with vigorous shaking (succussion).

➤ Raw materials, such as minerals, that are not soluble in water or alcohol are triturated or ground into fine powder before being mixed with a liquid.

➤ Homeopathic pharmacies apply the latest scientific and industrial standards to ensure safe and effective products.

➤ Homeopathic products are regulated by the FDA under the Federal Food, Drug, and Cosmetic Act of 1938.

➤ Homeopathic medicines can be purchased over-the-counter for self-limiting conditions and are exempt from expiration date requirements.

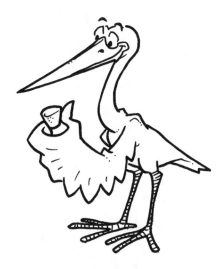

Chapter 6

Where Do Homeopathic Remedies Come From?

In This Chapter

➤ Discover the variety of sources used to make homeopathic products

➤ Learn how each family of medicines passes on its own distinct characteristics

➤ Find out how nature's bounty can help some common complaints

---

Wouldn't you like to have everything in your life customized so that it was just right? Who wouldn't want his favorite breakfast cooked just the way he likes it and all his clothing perfectly tailored? In homeopathic medicine, the goal of a practitioner is to customize your prescription so that the homeopathic medicine is as close to a perfect fit as possible. To accomplish this feat, homeopaths are constantly looking for new raw materials for proving so that the hidden message of the medicine may be used to help individuals who require this precise substance to achieve optimal health.

In this chapter, we'll take a look at of some of the well-known families of homeopathic medicines. Similar to your own family, this roundup of remedies has many more relatives than we have time to get to know. There are in-laws in our family who share properties of another family grouping; for instance, snake root plants belong to the plant kingdom while exhibiting many of the homeopathic signs of an animal remedy.

Your homeopath has studied long hours to learn how to distinguish which family of remedies will best suit your exact needs and which exception to the rules will customize your homeopathic prescription.

Minerals: Ironing Out the Edges

Minerals are the building blocks of our earth, and many components of our bodies are either made of or use minerals as a daily function of life. The mineral remedies in general help people who have issues around being organized—either too little, or too much.

The variations of minerals in terms of symptoms is as expansive as the 135 substances in the *Periodic Table of Elements*.

H Impulsive being																	He Being free: autism
Li Impulsive personality	Be Adapting person	B Doubting your personality							C A rigid or labile person					N Expansion of the ego: assertive	O Lost self-worth: begging	F Letting go of values: amoral	Ne Free from relations
Na Impulsive making and breaking relationships	Mg Looking for your place in the family	Al Confusion where you stand in relations							Si Obvious relations: family					P Sharing in relations: communication	S Deepening of relations: marriage	Cl Climax in relations: mother/child	Ar Free from work
K Simply doing your duty	Ca Observed in your job	Sc Scanning possible jobs	Ti Starting officially with work	V Doubting if you can do your job	Cr Proving that you can do your job	Mn Training your skills	Fe Persevering in your work	Co The last test for your skill	Ni Obvious control	Cu Keep your control: cramp	Zn Over-doing routines: repetition	Ga Retire to old routines	Ge Formal work: civil servant	As Loss of your job	Se Neglecting your work	Br Letting go of work:retire	Lr Free from performance
Rb Impulsive showing your artisticity	Sr Criticised on your ideas	Y Exploring creativity	Zr Starting your creative work	Nb Doubting your creative talents	Mo The challenge of the arts	Tc Training in creativity	Ru Forcing your inspiration	Rh Almost ready for your performance	Pd Obvious performance: actor	Ag Preserve the arts	Cd Repeating your creations	In Retire the old arts	Sn Discarded ideas and creations	Sb Loss of honor	Te Neglecting your creativity	I Letting go of culture	Xe Free from power
Cs Impulsive creating your power	Ba Power-less leader	La Searching for a leader position	Hf Starting as a manager	Ta Doubting if you can be a leader	W Prove your power	Re Training in managing	Os Force your power: crisis manager	Ir Almost the leader	Pt The obvious leader: king	Au Preserve the power	Hg Overdoing your power: tiranny	Tl Holding to old ways of managing	Pb Formal power diplomat	Bi Loss of leadership	Po Memories of power	At Letting go of power	Rn Free from magic

The Periodic Table of Elements *lists all the basic elements of our world. Jan Scholten (Scholten, 1996) has arranged and labeled them to reflect his experiences using them as homeopathic remedies.*

Ferrum Nitricum, a form of *iron,* is the mineral we'll look at closer. People who need Ferrum Nitricum as a homeopathic remedy tend to be firm, assertive, and push their way through work. They feel a great sense of duty and responsibility, which puts additional pressure on them to perform. They take great pride in their work and even the slightest criticism will provoke anger and unrest. Relaxation is a thing of the past and is only considered when satisfactory work has been accomplished. They are generally very disciplined people whose expectations of themselves are quite high.

Here are the basic symptoms calling for Ferrum Nitricum (Scholten, 1996):

➤ Fear of failure, criticism, enjoyment, strangers, future, crowds.

➤ Dreams of unsuccessful efforts, battles, fights, contests, falling, dead people.

➤ Most symptoms seem worse from being warm.

➤ Sleeplessness.

➤ Mental sluggishness.

➤ Redness, swelling, and experiencing a general or specific symptom of heat or fever.

➤ Hot flushes, worse at night.

➤ Headaches.

➤ Stomach complaints.

The professional homeopath will review all these symptoms and make sure that the remedy fits not only the physical complaint, but also the mental and emotional themes present. In this way, the prescriptions are completely customized and the greatest chance for a successful treatment is possible.

Menopause: Halting the Hormonal Heat

Irina was having difficulty with persistent night sweats that were keeping her from enjoying a restful sleep. This was important to Irina as she needed to perform her job as a scientist at one of the leading labs in my area. She was highly recognized throughout her industry and was a professor at a prestigious educational institution. She complained of hot flushes, dizzy spells, muddled thinking, and low energy. She had also recently been to see a gastroenterologist for stomach complaints: Nothing was found wrong. She was originally from the Ukraine, where she had her initial training as an engineer. "I believe in discipline, but lately I'm emotional. What can I do? You must help me. I don't give up!"

Irina began taking Ferrum Nitricum and, within a couple of weeks, began to feel better. After six weeks had passed, she was sleeping well, had energy, and was happily back at work.

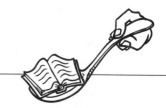

Dose of Info

Ferrum is the Latin name for **iron.** It's the fourth most common element on the earth and is the basic material for all forms of steel. It has historically been used in the precision manufacturing of both weapons and tools (Scholten, 1996).

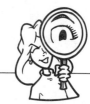

Curious Clues

Irina lived by order and discipline. The onset of menopause created a situation she could not control, and it was affecting the quality of the most important aspect of her self-worth: work and how she felt she was perceived. This situation combined with sleeplessness, hot flushes, and recent stomach complaints brought me to the remedy Ferrum Nitricum.

49

Plants: Nature's Tender Touch

The members of the plant kingdom are numerous and incredibly diverse. Their long history stretches back to the very development of earth, and land plants are thought to have colonized the shores of ancient seas some 400 million years ago. Scientists estimate that only about 300,000 species of plants have been classified. That may sound like a lot, but new species are being discovered and studied in our dwindling rain forests and remote corners of the globe. According to Wessell's and Kepson's text on biology, algae are the oldest plants on earth, showing a remarkable ability to thrive despite hardship. Algae have some dramatic changes on earth, but have been able to adapt and come out as the largest group of aquatic plants, and make up the greatest percentage of the earth's living organisms.

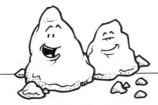

Natural Nuggets

Poison ivy, or *Rhus toxicodendron,* is listed in *The 2000 Edition of the Herbal Physician's Desk Reference* as causing "even in small amounts" severe irritation of the skin. Would you like more out of your ivy? Potentize it! The *Herbal Physician's Desk Reference* lists only homeopathic usage and treatment for this plant. When prepared according to homeopathic dilution and succussion (potentizing), the homeopathic medicine has been used to treat rheumatism in the joints and muscles, anxiety, depression, and irritated skin.

This ability or inability to adapt to life's challenges and insults, in a world "where they can only passively persist by developing adaptations," is at the center of understanding the homeopathic relationships in plant remedies (Wessell and Hopson, 1998). With such an enormous variety of plant life, you can well understand that your homeopath needs a great effort to understand the subtle relationships between the plant kingdom and all its families.

Asthma: Breathing Is Such Sweet Sorrow

Janice was down. She had not been feeling really "happy" for quite some time. She took her comforts privately with food. She worked in a restaurant where she could hide food during the evening, and when all the others had left, "I could eat my troubles away." She came into the office complaining of asthma, which had been getting worse ever since a new worker came to work during her shift. Her co-worker was bubbly and sociable. Janice had always been quiet, private, and withdrawn. She always wanted to be in a good relationship, but felt pestered every time a boyfriend was around. Her asthma had gotten worse when the "wowgirl" began work and Janice felt as if "everyone wanted me to be like her, not like myself."

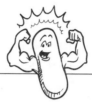

Potent Pellets

"Sequoia and pine are both familiar trees in the United States. People who need tree remedies in general feel hardness on the outside and fragile on the inside. They may have an inner feeling of being ugly. A homeopath may think generally of tree remedies, but most understand the subtle differences such as people who need sequoia feel unappreciated, feeling of pain around their heart, bladder, kidney, and lung problems. A pine remedy would help someone who felt he had to please others, yielding personality, feeling of being unloved, hay fever, nausea, and constipation. Both trees, two different kinds of patients to please."

Source: Louis Klein Master Class, 1995–1998

After a few doses of *Pseodotsusa*, or Douglas Fir, her asthma greatly improved. In about two months, she became less irritable at work and more tolerable of others. She saw the food addiction as an imbalance and began counseling. As the year progressed, she was able to become lighter, more cheery (which surprised her), and began to socialize more often. The food addictions and asthma were not an issue, and she had begun a relationship.

Animals: Survival Is the Name of the Game

You haven't eaten all day. Your stomach growls and knots up, reminding you of your neglected gastric duties. Suddenly it's become too much to bear. Your head pops up from your work, eyes flick quickly about your surroundings, focus becomes fixed on the object of your glare as you pounce on a piece of something to eat that never stood a chance. You're an animal! According to Helena Curtis, the author of *Biology*, you've exhibited the chief characteristic of animal survival, the hunting of prey, which requires efficient systems of integration and control. Instead of come and get it, animals go and get it.

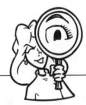

Curious Clues

What qualities or themes are important in this patient's story in order to select the homeopathic remedy Douglas Fir? Here are the ones I used in this particular case:

➤ Depressing quality

➤ Sensitive to criticism

➤ Unsocial, unplayful

➤ Feelings of unfulfilled relationships

➤ Food addictions, dreams of food, great food cravings

➤ Asthma

➤ Compulsive qualities that are hidden

➤ Desire for company, but aggravated when in company

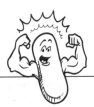

Potent Pellets

"Unlike plants, which are passive recipients of energy from the sun, animals must seek out food sources or alternate devise strategies for ensuring that the food comes to them. Mobility becomes an important instinct in animal survival" (Curtis, 1983).

The homeopathic remedy *Elaps* is made from the beautiful coral snake—remember the maxim "Red and yella, kill a fella"? Following the many thousands of dilutions it takes to become a homeopathic remedy, it is quite safe, and I've used it effectively to help many patients. Most people who would benefit from an animal remedy like Elaps display an aggressive nature. Elaps patients tend to be more manipulative than most with behavioral themes that include intolerance of contradiction, anxiety and fear. They may even suffer from panic attacks, which are usually more controlled in adults. According to homeopathic medical observations, patients who display animal characteristics— particularly people who would benefit from a snake remedy— enjoy adoring themselves with jewelry and dressing up. They often play the cute or sexy roles to the hilt.

Crocodile Tears ... It's Showtime!

Jenny was the life of the party until it was time for her to go to bed. This five-year old socialite would entertain a roomful of guests by parading around in Mom's dresses, hats, and jewelry. While in costume, she would sing songs, do skits, and ask people to give her their watches, jewelry, and money. She claimed her parents didn't give her enough lunch money. She had cravings for salads, had unexplained anxieties, and night terrors with dreams of dead friends and robbers. She was very pleasant if she was the center of attention, but would pout or cry if she was told to go to bed, or her will was contradicted in any way. I observed her several times turning her back on her mom while pretending to cry until she got her own way. She was in control of every vacation, dinner, and visit, or else!

The homeopathic remedy Elaps was able to help Jenny find balance in her personality. She began to listen more to her parents, have less of a showgirl attitude around others. She will probably always be outgoing, but she's finding a way to back off the intensity. Her unexplained fears and nightmares stopped, and her parents said she was easier to be with and take places.

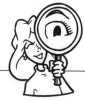

Curious Clues

Did you spot a snake in the grass? Here are some clues for prescribing Elaps (Klein, 1995–1998):

➤ Intolerant of contradiction

➤ Manipulative

➤ Desire to dress up in costumes and jewelry

➤ Dreams of the dead, robbers

➤ Anxiety

➤ Cravings for salads

➤ A feeling that someone is going to take what is theirs

Milk Remedies: Got Milk?

Milk is one of the universal nurturing substances we think of with a baby's first months of life. In fact, all mammals (animals that produce milk for their young) care for the initial stages of life with the energy and nutrition of milk. It's no wonder that homeopaths have potentized many different milks from a variety of mammals since the themes of nurturing and attachment are common in our society.

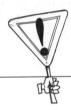

Caution Keeper

Homeopathic medicines are required by federal law to list one or two common indications on the side of the label. This listing is often misleading because of the many symptoms this remedy may help to heal if prescribed according to a full homeopathic match of the physical, mental, and emotional essence of the person to the remedy. Going by a single symptom often yields disappointing results. Find a qualified homeopath to help you sort out the choices.

People who could receive benefit from homeopathic milk remedies, if properly prescribed, would exhibit issues around nurturing or abandonment, a feeling of being forsaken, or breaking connections. This would be combined with other animalistic characteristics of aggression, a predatory behavior.

Lac Canium (*lac* means "milk," *canium* is "dog"), or dog's milk, combines the general qualities of milk remedies with the particular symptoms found when provers took the diluted homeopathic preparation. This remedy has been used for many years, and I have found it particularly effective for issues of self-esteem. The old saying, "They treated him like a dog," brings up many of the themes surrounding this time-tested homeopathic medicine. Individuals who may benefit from Lac Canium often have symptoms that include the effects of abuse or being tormented. They exhibit sensations of floating in air, depression, or lack of feeling. They experience dizziness, and women experience severe ovarian pain, which improves with the onset of menses. They often have a constant desire to urinate, which does not pass even after emptying the bladder. Painful swellings of the breasts and absent-mindedness can also be present to varying degrees.

Anger and Disappointment

Sally could make you smile in a heartbeat. Most of the time she forced herself to be upbeat, but complained of chronic depression. She came to see me about the severe ovarian pain she felt before her menses and the persistent fibrocystic breasts that caused her so much discomfort. She stated that she was a recovering alcoholic whose parents had also been alcoholics. She had raised herself because her mother was usually passed out on the sofa. She had difficulty holding down a job, because her mind wandered, and she would often float off in fantasy land. She had just gotten out of an abusive marriage and found herself full of shame, self-doubt, confusion and rage that erupted much more frequently than she wished. Lac Canium assisted Sally greatly in easing her burden. She was able to reach out for help, and dramatically lowered her physical and mental distress within a few months of taking the remedy.

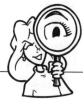

Curious Clues

Can you recognize the symptoms calling for Lac Canium?

➤ Angers easily

➤ History of neglect and abuse

➤ Severe ovarian pain, problems with menses

➤ Painful or fibrocystic breasts

➤ Sensations of floating

➤ Absent-mindedness

➤ Low self-esteem, depression

Herbs and homeopathics all start out the same. All raw material from the minerals or animal kingdom are collected and cleaned. Most of the time they are ground into fine powder or dissolved into a solution called a mother tincture. This is where the road forks. Herbal products stay in this form and are bottled or put into some other container or mixed with other herbs. Homeopathic medicines take the same substance and through a series of carefully monitored dilutions and succussion (shaking), increase the electromagnetic properties of the diluted solution creating—in time—a homeopathic or remedy medicine of the original substance.

I hope you've enjoyed your walk through the wild kingdom. Next we'll visit our own bodies and take a look at the principles of homeopathic prescribing.

The Least You Need to Know

➤ Mineral remedies help people who have issues around structure and organization, either too little or too much.

➤ Plant remedies assist individuals who are sensitive to their surroundings, passive, and adapt to being injured or hurt.

➤ Animal remedies match those who take what they want, are competitive, and have therapeutic themes for survival.

➤ Milk remedies can help your body to heal the wounds of abuse and neglect, for those overly irritated or angry.

Part 2

Symptoms and Simillimums

Symptoms are visible clues that give us an idea of what is going on inside of you. That's right, I said an idea! Even with the best diagnostic techniques available, no one can guarantee the diagnosis, prognosis, or result of treatment.

In this part of the book, you'll discover why homeopaths have become masters of observation, as well as the time-tested techniques and principles we use to choose a homeopathic medicine for you. You'll learn what a simillimum is and how it could be the key for healing your mind, body, and spirit.

The proof of treatment is always in the health of the patient. Homeopathy is uniquely suited to assist in the healing process both physically and mentally and for all ages. This part of the book demonstrates this concept by showing you some of the more common emotional conditions that can wreak havoc on your quality of life. We'll also take a look at pesky pediatric challenges for a different view of homeopathy's helpful therapies.

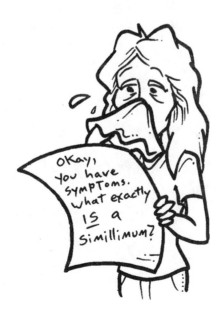

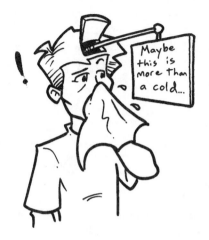

Chapter 7

The Principles of Homeopathy

In This Chapter

➤ Understand the importance of your vitality

➤ Examine the pillar of homeopathic prescribing: "like cures like"

➤ Discover why a minimal dose of medicine works

➤ Do you know what your body looks like when it heals?

You'll learn in this chapter that the vital force is a reliable indicator of how your body is coping with the stresses of disease. You'll see for yourself the principle theories and observations, such as Hering's directions of cure, that help homeopaths know how you're doing. "Like cures like" has been a theory; I will show you how it works with a patient.

We all want less pressure on us, fewer bills to pay, and fewer hours to work. What about less medicine? You'll learn how a minute or minimal dose of homeopathic medicine can jump-start your body's healing potential.

Vital Force: May the Force Be with You

We've all seen them. Perhaps you're one of them, the kind of person you can't ignore when they enter the room. They ooze with an unexplainable yet perceptible quality that we all recognize.

There are some people who bubble with life. The other end of the spectrum is also recognizable—people who seem lifeless. We don't know why, but we have a feeling when we're in their company that something is missing. These are only impressions, but it's not unusual for us to act on these instincts in our personal and business lives.

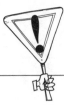

Caution Keeper

George Vithoulkas, a contemporary homeopathy practitioner in Greece, warns us that health depends on the strength of the vital force. He states, "This vital substance, when in a natural state, is constrictive; it keeps the body continuously constructed and reconstructed. But when the opposite is true, when the vital force from any cause withdraws from the body, we see that the forces that are in the body being turned loose are destructive" (Vithoulkas, 1980).

Early homeopaths were helping to heal the sick before the development of scientific processes and diagnostic equipment. They placed great value in helping to restore life quality or vital force to their patients. In *Organon of the Medical Art,* Samuel Hahnemann points out the difference between a healthy life force and one that is lacking this all-important quality. In Chapter 10 of his book he explains, "In the healthy human state, the spirit-like life force that enlivens the material organism, governs without restriction and keeps all parts of the organism in admirable, harmonious vital operation, as regards both feelings and functions, so that our indwelling, rational spirit can freely avail itself of this living, healthy instrument for the higher purposes of our existence" (O'Reilly, 1996).

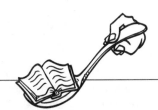

Dose of Info

According to John Ayto's *A Dictionary of Word Origins, vital* is an Old French word derived from the Latin *vitalis* or *vita* meaning "life, living, or capable of life." Force is the measure of your strength and vigor. They combine to form a key indicator for overall health in homeopathy. How is your **vital force?**

The principle of *vital force* reminds all of us that being alive is an ongoing process. The quality of life depends heavily on the presence of a strong and active vital force. This may at first sound like the immune system, but I can tell you it is much more. It combines the physical, mental, and emotional aspects of who we are as individuals with our dynamic interaction with our environment and all that surrounds us in an ever-changing world filled with challenges. A strong vital force is the key to being and staying healthy.

The Law of Similars

When Hahnemann found a better way to relieve suffering, he built his theories and the observations that have proved to be true throughout 200 years of homeopathy: *similia similibus curantur,* the Latin phrase meaning "let *similars* be cured by similars."

At the time, there was an abundance in medical practice of prescribing medicines according to the laws of dissimilars. If a patient was hot, give a medicine to cool him down; if there was pain, give something to take the pain away. Hahnemann saw that these treatments only covered up an illness, for if the medicine was stopped, the illness came back. No one was being truly helped, and often the side effects weakened the patient's vital force, which made it difficult for him to recover.

James Kent, a brilliant American homeopath practicing in the early 1900s, states in his book, *Lectures on Homeopathic Philosophy,* "after Hahnemann had made a number of provings, he gathered together from the literature a great number of reported cures for the purpose of observing whether the cures had been made accidentally or on purpose, and whether they were in accordance with the law of similars or with the principle of dissimilars. In every instance, he was able to see that the cures had been made in accordance with the law of similars" (Kent, 1979).

Over the last two centuries, homeopaths have continued to follow the law of similars because it works. When I am able to correctly match the symptoms of a patient with these symptoms produced by a healthy person in a homeopathic proving, the results are tremendous. The patient begins to improve in all ways and feels his overall health and vitality return. The old symptoms do not come back; there are no side effects, and the patient does not have to stay on the medicine in order to continue feeling well. We study therapeutic principles

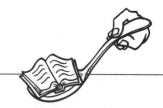

Dose of Info

The Latin phrase *similia similibus curantur*—"let **similars** be cured by similars"—is often translated as *like cures like.* This refers to the principle of effectively treating diseases that Samuel Hahnemann made popular in the late 1700s. He found that medicines that were able to cure a patient's illness would also produce "similar" symptoms of this illness when given in minute doses to a healthy person.

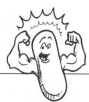

Potent Pellets

Until the late 1840s, French physicians had the right to perform the autopsy of their dead patients so that the connection between the symptoms and possible cause of death could be better understood. Despite a growing amount of medical knowledge, diseases were still thought to be from an imbalance of humors, treated primarily through purging by bleeding or inducing vomiting, sweating, or diarrhea.

and search for the best homeopathic remedy whose provers had similar symptoms as our patient. In this way, the body is strengthened, and illness can be overcome.

Minimum Dose: One Station at a Time

Have you ever tried to understand what was being played on a radio station that was in between two stations? You catch pieces of both but not enough to really comprehend either one. It's confusing and frustrating. In contrast, when you're finally tuned into the station that helps you carry that particular mood, it's so very satisfying. When properly prescribed by homeopathic principles, homeopathy is like that. Patients receive one remedy at a time. One minute dose of a substance that the practitioner feels the body can "listen to," and the inner wisdom of the vital force will understand enough to begin the healing process. Since a well-chosen remedy is tuned into the same frequency or station as the patient, the match will result in strengthening the patient's natural healing abilities. Matching the individual frequency is a key process that means the difference between nothing happening and stimulating our vital force to heal.

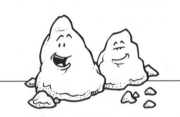

Natural Nuggets

According to the Society of Homeopaths, the law of similars (like cures like) principle of homeopathy is often compared to vaccinations. Vaccines introduce a small amount of the weakened virus or bacterium related to a disease into the body in order to raise the body's immune response against that disease. Homeopathic remedies are extremely diluted and therefore no diseased materials (biological or chemical) are introduced into the body.

As you've learned, homeopathic medicines are greatly diluted substances that have no threat of side effects or addiction. Since we are looking for an energetic solution to healing, there is no need to force chemical reactions in your body to receive health. The dynamic diluted solutions you read about in Chapter 1, "What Is Homeopathy and How Does It Work?" hold far greater electromagnetic potential than nonhomeopathic solutions.

Some of the greatest moments in my career have come from listening to a skeptical person as he leaves my office say, "Is this all you're going to give me?" and having him on a follow-up visit say, "It's amazing how that little bit of something helped me so much!" We're trained by advertisers to think more is better. Remember the first time you opened up a gigantic box of cereal and found only a relatively small portion in the box? Looks can be deceiving. With homeopathy, a carefully chosen remedy can assist your body's innate ability to heal. Samuel Hahnemann said it best, "The only calling of a physician is to cure rapidly, gently, and permanently."

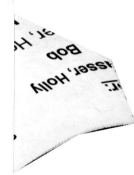

A Tickling Cough

Jane was an old romantic. She wrote special love notes and tucked them into her husband's coats, briefcase, and lunch bag. She would wait for his call at work and swoon in her chair, saying, "My knight in shining armor is on the line." The winter had begun, and Jane had developed a chronic tickling cough that was worse when she came from outdoors to inside her heated office. Her nose was often blocked up at work where she thought the room temperature was too hot. She didn't like to be hot. She was quite overweight, soft, and sensitive. Although she came into the clinic for her cough, she also complained about many gastrointestinal complaints such as poor digestion, hiccups, and nausea, especially if she went off her diet. Her bowels often alternated between diarrhea and constipation.

I gave her Antimonium Crudum, which not only resolved the cough within a few days, but eventually helped her find relief from the numerous gastro complaints.

The principle of the minimum dose allows a homeopath to give you the smallest possible amount of a remedy that will still gently, yet effectively, elicit a reaction from your body's vital force so that healing can begin.

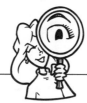

Curious Clues

See if you recognize the general or unusual symptoms that pointed me toward Antimonium Crudum (Morrison, 1993):

➤ Quiet, soft, sensitive, and emotional.

➤ Often described as "mellow and romantic in the moonlight."

➤ General aggravation from radiant heat such as stove, heater, or open fire.

➤ Nasal obstruction, worse from heat.

➤ Cough entering a warm room.

➤ Chronic, tickling cough.

➤ Weak digestion.

➤ Nausea, worse from poor diet.

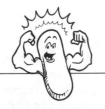

Potent Pellets

When looking at the total symptom picture of a patient, the goal of every homeopath is to find the simillimum. The simillimum remedy, which is different for every person, is the closest match between what the provers of the remedy experienced and the patient's symptoms. It is the most similar to what the patient is experiencing and will do the most good for the patient's health.

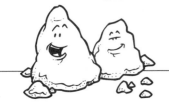

Natural Nuggets

Keeping a diary or journal where you jot down changes to your condition, noting interesting and unusual sensations that you experience, is a great way to accurately inform your homeopath of your progress. Most office visits are four to eight weeks apart; so keep it fresh in your mind by writing it down.

Hering's Direction of Cure: A Road Map for Remedies

Now you see it, now you don't. That's how things disappear in a magic show. While homeopathic treatment can yield some seemingly magical results, in chronic conditions it is often the skill of evaluating the progression of health that clarifies the action of the remedy. These evaluations usually combine the story that the patient relates to you along with a homeopath's experience at gauging subtle changes while gaining an understanding of the patient's advance or retreat from illness.

When a patient has been given the correct homeopathic remedy that stimulates the body's vital force toward healing, there are repeatable and observable symptoms that improve in particular order. Generally, symptoms go from the more essential functions of the body to less essential areas.

Pediatric eczema and asthma are prime examples of the direction of cure that I see too frequently in my clinic. I will often see children with these difficult problems. Their medical histories are shockingly similar. The child is usually born with eczema and is prescribed a conventional topical medication that clears up the eczema. Within one or two months, the child develops bronchitis, is treated with more medications, and eventually is diagnosed as having asthma. The child must now rely heavily on medications to breathe and might even be limited athletically.

Follow the bouncing pellets as we discuss the direction of cure. After the child has taken the correct homeopathic medicine, the first organs that are likely to begin improving are the lungs. Asthma can be a debilitating condition that breeds fear and hesitation in many young developing children. As the vital force is stimulated, breathing improves (more vital to less vital), and asthma may revert back to symptoms those children had before their asthma diagnosis (in reverse order). As healing progresses, the lungs feel much improved, and to everyone's surprise the eczema returns (from inside out). With continued treatment, the eczema is gone and so is the asthma, and the child behaves in a freer, more confident manner.

Even with all of the scientific technology and innovative diagnostic tests and therapies available, it is often experienced judgment based on discerning observations that leads us to place our trust in health-care practitioners. This chapter has included some of the homeopathic principles that have been tested, observed, and retested over two centuries by dedicated practitioners in search of the simillimum. Our process continues in the next chapter as we go one on one and see what it's like to go to your first homeopathic visit.

The Least You Need to Know

➤ Your health depends on the strong and harmonious functions of your vital force.

➤ The law of similars states that medicines that were able to cure a patient's illness would also produce "similar symptoms" of that illness when given in minute doses to a healthy person.

➤ Homeopathic medicines are prescribed one at a time.

➤ The principle of the minimum dose allows a homeopath to give the smallest possible amount of a remedy that will still elicit a healing reaction.

➤ Hering's direction of cure enables a homeopath to gauge the progress of a patient's condition based on the course or direction the illness takes in your body.

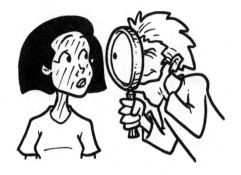

Chapter 8

Your First Visit to a Homeopath

In This Chapter

➤ Find out what to expect on your first visit to a homeopath

➤ Learn why getting the total picture of a patient is key to finding the best remedy

➤ Physical, mental, and emotional symptoms are important

➤ Discover the tools of the trade your homeopath uses

➤ Understand the difference between homeopathy and homeotherapies

Remember being invited to a friend's home for dinner and asking, "What can I bring?" and your friend saying, "Just bring yourself." That is exactly the most important element to bring to your first homeopathic visit. I certainly welcome lab reports and diagnostic narratives so that I understand the disease state or injury as thoroughly as possible. However, the field of homeopathy recognizes that this condition exists in the most unique and particularly individual environment: you! Symptoms are your body's best attempt at healing itself. They are an indication of how your own system is dealing with this condition at this moment. As you change, so do the symptoms.

I'll take you through the components of your first visit so that you can get some idea of what kinds of confirmation your homeopath wants to know. I can honestly tell you that you already know all the answers. I'll show you the way we look at your symptoms, how we organize the ideas, and why those "funny little sensations" you feel may be a clue to your condition.

Wonder what we do with all that info? You'll see for yourself how a practitioner peruses through the pages or clatters on the keyboard searching for the best remedy. Do you know the difference between homeopathy and homeotherapies? Soon you'll discover which one is right for you.

Listening and Learning

New patients are often surprised that I've set aside between one and two hours to listen to their story. When we get seated, I usually ask, "How may I help you?" What typically follows is a description of the condition that motivated the patient to make an appointment. I initially let the patient determine the direction of our discussion.

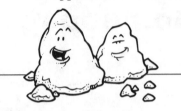

Natural Nuggets

Patients are surprised when I don't bombard them with questions but instead ask, "Is there anything else?" Then I can observe all the qualities of their state of being as they spontaneously occur. Is there spontaneity, clarity, or intensity in what they say? When do they gain energy and excitement or become quiet or refuse to discuss things further? With proper listening and practice, I can recognize these qualities.

I'm open to listening and understanding the condition and the state of the patient's health in whatever aspects she feel are important. This openness allows a freedom that is rarely experienced in today's medical environment.

There is time for your story to unfold. Your homeopath will actively listen and pay a keen level of attention to what you are saying. As the visit progresses, your practitioner will begin to interpret what you have said and how you have said it in order to begin the process of choosing the most appropriate remedy.

Homeopaths also write down what you say. In this way, we get your own words to describe your condition and will bring your case alive when we study it. The purpose is to match as closely as possible the patient's total symptom picture with the provers' remedy picture. A homeopathic practitioner does not tell you why you do the things you do or counsel you on your behavior. That is left up to mental health professionals who are trained in emotional counseling, just as we have skills in choosing homeopathic remedies. Your own words are the key to understanding.

Modalities: For Better or for Worse?

Modalities are usually the causes or situations in which you generally, or your symptoms specifically, feel better or worse. For instance, Spigelia, a homeopathic remedy, may be a good match for someone who experiences chest pain on the left side of the body that is made worse from motion or inhaling, while being better from warm drinks. In homeopathy, we take information or sensations that you feel and use that as a guide to help find a remedy.

Modalities help us categorize some of your important experiences. The following table lists characteristics of frequently reoccurring, strong symptoms. A patient who would benefit from the homeopathic remedy Dioscorea may experience some or all of these symptoms:

Modalities Dioscorea (Homeopathic Wild Yam)

Better from

Open air

Elevating feet helps lower-back pain

Lying down aids pain in the lungs

Exercise feels good for legs

Lying down on back and pulling hair in front of ears benefits colic

Worse from

Getting cool aggravates knee pain

Inhalation creates dizziness

Motion increases pain on the left side of the chest

Sitting up in bed increases all pain

Eating stimulates pain around the navel

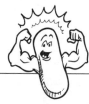

Potent Pellets

All of a patient's symptoms can be described under different categories that combine to form one picture (Sankaran, 1994):

➤ Pace of speech

➤ Sensitivity or excitability to food, environment, emotions, and so on

➤ State of mind and dreams

➤ Nature of the illness and its meaning to the patient

➤ Causation—how did this all start, is it an acute or chronic condition

➤ Genetic or inherited considerations

➤ Past history

Chronic Tonsillitis: Tormented Tonsils

Everyone knew to be gentle around Julie. She was extremely shy and would cling to her mom or wedge her seven-year-old body under a chair that her mother was sitting on. Julie was coming in for a homeopathic consultation for the chronic inflammation of her tonsils. She had been prone to getting sick with a stuffed-up nose and always a sore throat. "She refused to speak up in the office," her mom said. "Julie complained that she felt like a ball was stuck in her throat." It made it difficult to swallow. Cold drinks helped with the soreness of her throat, but she still had enlarged tonsils that her physician said needed to come out. Her parents often didn't know when her throat hurt, because Julie rarely spoke up at home. She struggled with going to school and lacked much of the confidence to keep going through her difficulties. She needed coaxing and reassurance to continue new activities.

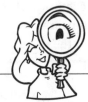

Curious Clues

Can you pick out the symptoms that would be helped by Baryta Muricatica (Morrison, 1993)?

➤ Acute or chronic tonsillitis

➤ Enlarged tonsils feel better with cold drinks

➤ Sensation of a lump in the throat that prevents swallowing

➤ Nasal obstruction

➤ Lack of self-confidence

➤ Extreme shyness, hides behind her mother

➤ Desire for reassurance

➤ Great difficulty with schoolwork

➤ School phobias

Julie was given Baryta Muricatica because the total symptoms she experienced, both physical and emotional, matched the symptoms of the provers of this remedy. As she began to experience a decrease in throat pain and discomfort, she also began to explore her surroundings without as much fear. She eventually became free of all swelling in her tonsils without any noticeable reoccurrence. Her surgery was canceled. Julie also began to interact more with her classmates and became more comfortable speaking up in class and doing schoolwork. She became more sociable and independent from her mother. In this way, prescribing all of her symptoms, Julie could gain freedom in her physical, mental, and emotional life, thus living her life more fully.

Surveying Your Symptoms

Symptoms are your body's best attempt at doing its own self-healing. These are the visible occurrences that we can see or experience. They are an important part of finding the correct homeopathic remedy. It was the formation of *symptoms* that was recorded by the healthy individuals who did proving experiments on all the remedies. We now match your symptoms with the proving symptoms in choosing the most helpful remedy.

Your homeopathic practitioner will be reviewing the symptoms that motivated you to make the appointment. As we discussed earlier, it will also be equally important to review your health history in regard to any physical or emotional feelings that are concerning or limiting you.

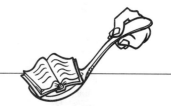

Dose of Info

The word **symptom** has not always been associated with signs of disease. It originally was part of everyday Greek language: *sumptoma* (occurrence) is a derivative of *sumpiptein,* which means *fall on* or *happen to.*

Physical Symptoms: Oh My Achin' Back!

Being a homeopathic practitioner would be such an easy job if you came in complaining of lower-back pain, and I said, "Ah yes, the homeopathic back remedy!" Currently I count more than 515 remedies that can help back pain.

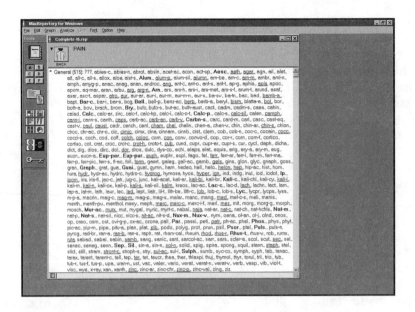

More than 515 homeopathic remedies may help back pain. Computer software, such as MacRepertory from Kent Homeopathic Association, helps homeopaths organize and compare enormous volumes of information. Remedy names are abbreviated and coded according to standard homeopathic convention. Bold type means that back pain was a strong and frequent experience of the provers; underlining means the pain was slightly less felt; plain type means even fewer provers indicated back pain as part of their experience. The feature options to the left of the screen organize, store, and search for symptoms; look up key words; and build graphs to continue the process of selecting the most accurate and effective homeopathic remedy.

(Source: Kent Homeopathic Associates)

What's next? Now we match the physical complaints with your individual experience. Does your back bother you only in the morning when you get out of bed? Does your lower back ache when you move, cough, breathe, or only before your menses? All of these specific answers help to narrow down the choices of a remedy.

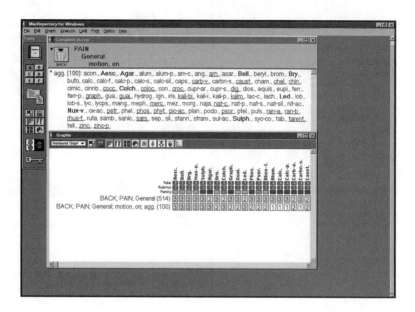

*Modalities individualize your choices of a remedy. When does your back pain get better and what makes it worse? Our choices have gone from 515 to 100 by indicating back pain felt with motion. The top section of MacRepertory shows the abbreviated homeopathic remedy choices, with the convention of bold, underlining, and plain type showing the frequency of this symptom in a proving. The lower section allows a homeopath to compare remedies in a graph. Symptoms are on the left while the remedies, in order of strength during a proving, are on top. The graph indicates the total number of rubrics. A remedy appears along with the family—plant, mineral, or animal. (The program is color-coded but is shown in black and white here.) The numbers in the boxes match the word convention above. For example, Bryonia is in the top row, right-hand corner, in bold type—**Bry.** On the graph, Bryonia is listed as the third remedy along the top, and the number 3 in the boxes corresponds to the bold typing for both symptoms.*

(Source: Kent Homeopathic Associates)

The modalities will further help in narrowing down your remedy choice. When does your back get better and what makes it worse?

Modalities of lower-back pain. Describing when it's better and what makes it worse helps match your individual experience with the findings of a prover and narrows down the remedy choices. If your homeopath enters vital symptoms key to your case, he or she can expect to find an appropriate remedy in this graph.

(Source: Kent Homeopathic Associates)

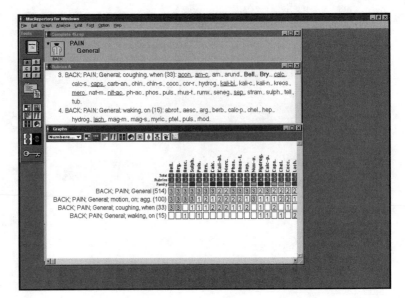

Clarity and intensity are vital components in using a particular symptom to select a remedy. Your homeopath must be clear that the physical symptoms that are being used are important and strong components to your complaints. After we've gotten straight on your physical symptoms, it's time to look at other aspects of you. After all, you're not just a back.

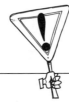

Caution Keeper

James Kent, a famous homeopath, reminds us to treat every person uniquely when he writes, "It is a great mistake for anyone to fit remedies for complaints or states. It is a fatal error for the physician to go on the bedside of a patient with the feeling in his mind that he has had cases similar to this one," thinking, "In the last case I had I gave so and so, therefore I will give it to this one." This is a clear warning for us to avoid lazy shortcuts by taking great care in intently listening to each individual patient (Kent, 1979).

The Strain of Emotional Pain

After a while, most of your friends and family do not want to hear in-depth how you feel. We do! Your emotions can be an extremely helpful part of the whole picture of your health. Homeopathy can treat a wide variety of conditions, including many of the mental and emotional complaints that detract from the quality of your life. Just as in the physical symptoms, your homeopath will want to listen to you describe your situation and will determine what is the most limiting symptoms you talk about that may lead us to the best remedy choice.

I remember one patient who came in complaining of a chest cold and had described himself as Eeyore in *Winnie the Pooh.* He said his depression and sadness lay on him like a heavy winter coat. No matter what else he did that day, he felt as if that heavy, bulky coat was wearing him down all day.

As we spoke, it became apparent to me that the frequent coughs motivated the patient to make the appointment, but the constant feeling of heavy sadness was limiting the vital force from helping to heal. This became an important clue for selecting the homeopathic remedy.

The patient was eventually given Causticum, which resolved the cough satisfactorily. Homeopathic treatment will help the patient to take off that old heavy winter coat (a metaphor for sadness) and allow joy and lightness to be a part of his life.

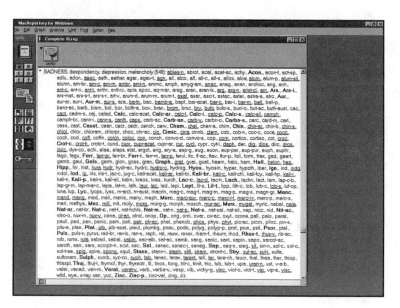

The list of homeopathic remedies that may help sadness or depression narrows the search down to 548. While sadness may be the most obvious complaint, homeopaths must be more specific about the person's individual experience to select the exact appropriate homeopathic remedy.

(Source: Kent Homeopathic Associates)

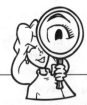

Curious Clues

Homeopaths find that dreams, or your feelings associated with dreams, are helpful because so many of the proving symptoms of homeopathic remedies have reported dreams. These are repetitive themes in dreams that are new to the individual. Often dreams represent feelings that we may have during the day, but our busy lives or medications often hide them from our attention. Children will many times not be able to describe their feelings, but can vividly recount recent dreams. Homeopaths don't interpret dreams, but use them to match up to the best remedy for their patients. I am continually surprised by the number of dreams that have been studied and listed in the homeopathic repertory. Here are a few examples of dreams and some of the remedies associated with them:

➤ Adventure: baryta carbonicum, ozone, sulphur

➤ Sadness: aluminum, arsenicum, naturum-muriaticum, pulsatilla

➤ Battle: allium cepa, bamboo, bayonia, hyosimus, naturum suphuricum, platinum

➤ Pursued by a witch that creeps under the door: ozone

➤ Being pinched: phosphorus

➤ Religion: hydrogen, kali muriaticum, sol-t-ae, sulphur

➤ Robbers: aluminum, naturum muriaticum, magnesium carbonicum, zinc

➤ Fire: anacardium, hepar sulphuricum, magnesia carbonica

➤ Ghosts: argentums nitricum, camphor, carbo vegatalis, graphitis, kali carbonica

Strange, Rare, and Peculiar Symptoms

When I first studied homeopathy, there were symptoms that I thought were so far-fetched that I would never hear in practice. Then I had a patient describing his condition. He stopped, looked at me, and said, "I know this sounds strange, but I always feel as if I have a loose hair across the tip of my tongue. I often wipe my tongue, but there is nothing there." This unusual sensation has been recorded time after time by healthy individuals who participate in the homeopathic proving of silicae. I took the rest of the case history, and since the totality fit silicae, I gave this as my remedy choice. The condition did resolve satisfactory. The unusual sensation that was given spontaneously and felt strongly by the patient became a core clue to the case.

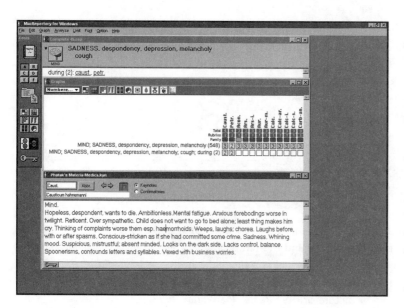

The MacRepertory software enables homeopaths to quickly and accurately select key individual or unusual characteristics to match with a remedy. While a computer does not make the selection, these programs can direct practitioners to additional information about a remedy under consideration, for example, in a materia medica, which may lead to a decision about using the homeopathic Causticum.

(Source: Kent Homeopathic Associates)

Over the years, I've found that patients do have these unusual experiences. When I look them up, I most often find that they have also been felt by healthy individuals during a homeopathic proving. Many of the consistent symptoms that patients clearly and strongly experience can be significant in helping their homeopath in selecting the best remedy for them.

Here are some examples of strange, rare, and peculiar symptoms:

➤ Anacardium: Sensation of a blunt plug stuck in a location in the body (joints, stomach, and so on).

➤ Antimonium Tartaricum: Overwhelming sleepiness during a cough or bronchitis.

➤ Arum Triphyllum: Constantly biting lips or picking them with fingers, may cause bleeding.

➤ Equistam: More urging to urinate when the bladder is empty, less urging when the bladder is full.

➤ Hydrophobinum: Generally feel worse from hearing the sound of running water.

➤ Ignatia: Sensation of a lump in the throat.

Tools of the Trade

The information that your homeopath must sift through while choosing your remedy is extensive. For each symptom there are usually many possible remedies. Narrowing down the choices involves finding the main concerns and selecting the remedies that fit the *totality of symptoms* including any strange or unusual ones that are more indicative of a single remedy.

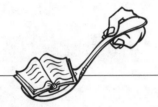

Dose of Info

Homeopaths match the picture of the patient's **totality of symptoms** with the picture of the remedy. "The essential idea behind the term totality of symptoms is that all the signs and symptoms present in an individual at a time arise from one basic disturbance which is the disease of the individual. When all the symptoms are put together, they become a meaningful form or picture of the disease" (Sankaran, 1994).

The tools that a homeopath has are the *Materia Medica* and the repertory. The *Materia Medica* is a dictionary of homeopathic medicines and their symptoms, and is the final authority on homeopathy. The *Materia Medica* contains the list of symptoms experienced by provers of the medicine, with the symptoms arranged in a systematic order.

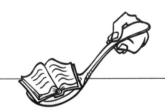

Dose of Info

A **repertory** is a list of things "found." The word is derived from late Latin *repeatorium,* which means *to find out.* The word was later used in nineteenth-century French as *repertoire,* meaning a list of plays, music, or performances.

The repertory is an index to the *Materia Medica.* This book contains all possible symptoms arranged in alphabetical order for each of the organs of the body. The practitioner has to regularly refer to this book to find out the medicines that have produced the symptoms of the patient in a prover. Your practitioner may have a set of books or a laptop computer next to him. If he starts typing on the computer or flipping through pages of a book, it means he's still listening to you and has begun to think of a specific remedy or family of remedies.

Repertory: The First Filter

When listening to symptoms, your homeopath may use the *repertory,* which classifies symptoms according to location of your body such as mind, head, stomach, back, abdomen, and so on.

Each symptom has the homeopathic remedies that are associated with it. Each remedy is graded as to the frequency and intensity of a particular symptom that the provers experienced while proving the remedy. Usually this is done by way of printing the letters. Bold type means this symptom was strongly experienced by most provers, while italicized lettering was felt less often, and plain type was experienced the least frequently by the provers.

The more specific information your homeopath gets the better. Patients say, for instance, "I'd like you to give me the homeopathic remedy for asthma." While being a condition, asthma is too general to narrow down a remedy choice. By my last count using MacRepertory, a computerized repertory, there are 348 remedies that have some effect on asthma.

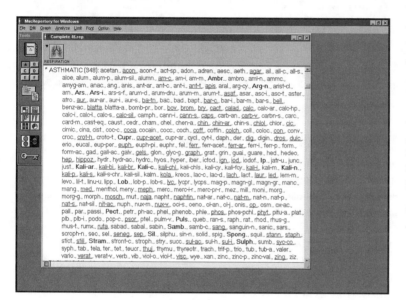

New patients will often say, "Give me the homeopathic remedy for asthma." According to the repertory, a homeopath has a choice of 348 remedies. To find the most effective remedy, homeopaths must look closer and find unique characteristics that reflect the whole person.

(Source: Kent Homeopathic Associates)

What is now needed is to get the particulars of the asthma, when is it better, worse, how did it begin, do you experience asthma along with any other symptoms? Your answers will further define the asthma which can be looked up more specifically in the repertory so that we can narrow down the remedy choices even further.

Your homeopath will classify the most important symptoms and narrow the choices to a few remedies. Then it's time to read about the remedies in order to select the best choice. For this we will need to choose one of the materia medicas.

By using rubrics that reflect the total picture of the patient as well as important individual characteristics, we narrowed our choices down to 21 remedies. From here, it's time to read about these remedies in a materia medica, which shows all the proving symptoms listed by system (mind, lung, stomach, etc.). This process allows homeopaths to study the remedy to make a careful choice.

(Source: Kent Homeopathic Associates)

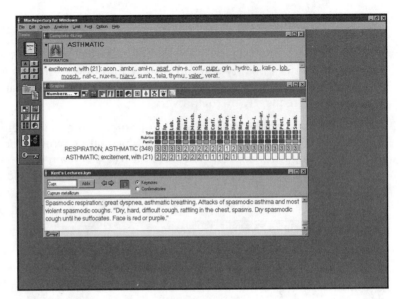

Materia Medica: Perusing the Provings

Medical matter or "materia medica" are the records of the homeopathic provers' symptoms usually categorized in the same format as the repertory (mind, head, back, abdomen, skin, and so on). You can use the repertory to select a few remedy possibilities, and then read the materia medica before making your final selection. I speak of this as if it might be one great book, when in fact over the centuries there have been many outstanding versions of materia medicas. Since Hahnemann's time, homeopaths have been writing their medical knowledge of the remedies they have used to pass on to their profession. There are many materia medicas to choose from which reflect the times and experience of their authors.

I use a laptop computer so that I may jump from one to another as I select the author who I may have trained with or one whom I believe has the most accurate proving records of a remedy. Jan Scholten is highly regarded for his work on understanding the mineral homeopathic remedies. I will often look at his book of materia medica to see if the patient I am trying to match the remedy with has the same symptoms as the mineral I'm thinking of.

The use of materia medica, which is being added to all the time by new provings, is an essential component to the selection of a homeopathic remedy by examining the totality of the symptoms. The more precise, unusual, or particular the symptoms are, the greater the possibility that the chosen remedy will match the patient's experience and healing will be initiated. Take the time to develop your knowledge and trust that correctly prescribed remedies work well.

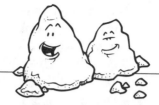

Natural Nuggets

Homeopathy is a wonderful medical art that can be practiced effectively at many levels of knowledge. Knowing your limits is important. Find a beginner's course to take or join a homeopathic study group in your area. To find the groups and courses, ask for assistance of a homeopath in your area, or call the National Center for Homeopathy or Homeopathic Educational Services, both listed in Appendix E, "Homeopathic Schools." They will assist you in finding the group or course that best matches your experience and desired level of study.

Homeopathy vs. Homeotherapies

I hear the word *homeopathic* used in many sales and marketing products. The general public associates the term with safe and effective. I'm concerned that this word will come to be so abused that it will resemble the term *natural*. I used to know what natural meant, but when I see it used on cereal and potato chip bags, I get confused. Show me a potato chip tree or bush!

The entire book so far has been discussing homeopathic principles of finding the exact remedy to match the totality of the patient's symptoms with the prover's symptoms. I've outlined the specific homeopathic manufacturing principles and standards in Chapter 5, "How to Make a Homeopathic Remedy." We've discussed the labor-intensive manner in which homeopathy is practiced in taking the time to listen and understand the true limitations that hold a patient back from a healthy fulfilling life. This is homeopathy.

This practice of *homeotherapeutics* combines several homeopathic remedies of low strength that have similar abilities to help a symptom. You can see these marketed to you in health food stores with easy-to-recognize names such as "cough," "PMS," or "allergy." These are designed to give you the confidence to self prescribe and buy the product

Dose of Info

Homeotherapeutics is a group of practices that use homeopathic dilutions of a substance, but do not necessarily comply with the same FDA regulations as homeopathy does. They also differ in that the homeopathics may be mixed together in what is commonly called a combination remedy.

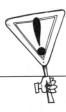

Caution Keeper

I've met many patients who say, "I've tried homeopathy; it doesn't work!" Many times what they've tried are over-the-counter homeotherapeutic products like "dry cough" or "sore throat." Later they were happy they tried it again using sound homeopathic principles of searching for the simillimum. Find a qualified homeopath near you if you are dissatisfied with the results of homeotherapeutic products.

for your condition. If you look on the side of the box, you'll see several remedies that are usually at 6x, 9x, or 6c strengths. This is a shotgun approach to homeopathy, hoping that one of these remedies may effectively control your symptoms.

You may see products marketed as homeopathic soap, shampoo, or homeopathic remedies combined with vitamins, herbs, or even conventional pharmaceuticals. Know that this is not the classical form of homeopathy that we have been discussing in this text. However, this is certainly a way to introduce products and awareness to the general public.

Homeotherapeutic products may even help some people get particular symptoms under control who do not have severe or chronic conditions. They are also the subject of several medical studies using them to treat specific conditions and have a tradition of being used widely in some countries. However they are not typically prescribed using the thorough interview and analysis approach to make a match with the total health picture of the patient. The patients' stories of complete healing that you will read about in the rest of this book have come from using classical homeopathic practices and single remedies, not the combinations typically seen in homeotherapeutic products.

James Kent said, "Science is knowledge and the application of knowledge is the art." Homeopathy is a medical art that combines all the practitioner's knowledge of medicine and healing with the skills of listening and subtle discernment. Keeping yourself centered, balanced, and attentive while serving the needs of a suffering patient is truly an art form, and one that homeopaths have to continue perfecting each day.

In the next chapter, we're going right into the emotional states of anxiety, depression, grief, and other experiences that if overdone can be a burden to your soul. Follow along with me, and I'll show you the hope that homeopathy can give.

The Least You Need to Know

➤ Careful and patient listening is an essential quality for obtaining a full and complete understanding of a patient's history.

➤ Discovering the "totality of symptoms" enables the homeopath to know what needs to be healed.

➤ Knowing the modalities of symptoms helps to narrow down the choices in prescribing a remedy.

➤ Symptoms may be physical, mental, or emotional. The more accurate and particular the symptoms, the greater the likelihood of choosing the best remedy.

➤ A repertory helps you to narrow down remedies by symptoms.

➤ A materia medica enables you to choose a final homeopathic medicine by carefully examining the proving symptoms of a remedy.

➤ While homeopathy employs the principle of using a single remedy for the totality of symptoms, homeotherapeutic products combine several low-strength remedies with other substances in hope that this shotgun approach will help control your symptoms.

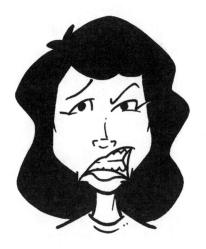

Chapter 9

Mental and Emotional Conditions

In This Chapter

➤ Learn how homeopathic medicines can end your anxious moments

➤ Discover the peace of mind homeopathic remedies offer for panic attacks and nightmares

➤ Find out the possibilities of relief from grief

➤ Break the cycle of depression with homeopathic remedies

If your arm is in a sling, or there's a bandage wrapped around your head, everyone can see you're not feeling well. If you get up out of a chair hobbling with stiff joints, most of us will offer help or take the cue not to push you to go hiking over the weekend. With mental and emotional conditions, there's nothing to see, and with social stigmas against being labeled "crazy," most people suffer in silence.

According to Dr. David Rosen of *Health News,* a recent surgeon general's report revealed that mental disorders will affect half of us at some point in our lives. These symptoms are still viewed as a personal weakness instead of a medical condition and nearly two-thirds of people who suffer from emotional conditions go untreated. Do you share with anyone the everyday struggles that feel like you're pushing a big rock uphill? Help is on the way!

The conditions you're going to read about permeate almost every aspect of the patients' lives that are being shared with you. In this chapter, you'll see how some of the most debilitating emotional conditions such as anxiety, panic attacks, and nightmares can be effectively treated using homeopathic medicines.

Generalized Anxiety Disorder

Excessive daily worry or restlessness lasting for more than six months about a number of activities or events is how the *Merck Manual* defines *generalized anxiety disorder* (*GAD*). Usually there's nothing specific that is bugging you, just a general uneasy feeling that you can't shake off. Sometimes the sensations become so strong that you have to limit your activities in order to remain somewhat calm.

Here are the symptoms of GAD:

➤ Excessive worry

➤ Restlessness

➤ Difficulty concentrating, confusion

➤ Startled easily

➤ Irritable

➤ Feeling wound up tight

➤ Fatigue

➤ Shortness of breath

➤ Palpitations

➤ Dry mouth

➤ Nausea, diarrhea

➤ Sleep problems

➤ Excessive urinating, frequency or urgency

➤ Sweaty or clammy skin

➤ Dizziness

➤ Unexpected flushing or chills

Dose of Info

GAD or **generalized anxiety disorder** affects 3 percent to 5 percent of the U.S. population within a one-year period. Women are twice as likely to be affected as men. GAD often begins in childhood or adolescence, but may begin at any age. Common worries include work responsibility, money, health, safety, car repairs, and household chores.

Source: The Merck Manual, 17th Edition

Anxiety disorders are the most common of all mental conditions, and research suggests that GAD may run in families. Sometimes the anxiety coexists with depression, substance abuse, or other disorders such as panic attacks, irritable bowel syndrome, headaches, or insomnia. People with GAD find it difficult to relax, often have uncontrolled feelings of impending disaster, or something they have left undone. I've had patients describe the feeling as being on red alert about everything.

Treatment with conventional medicines includes the use of benzodiazepines, although sustained use can cause physical dependence. Other medications such as Buspinore and antidepressants are also being researched and used for this type of anxiety. Behavioral therapy yields limited benefits, according to the *Merck Manual,* because there are no specific anxiety triggers to address. Biofeedback and relaxation techniques may offer some individuals help with stress and muscle relaxation.

Anxiety: Perception Deception

Jack was a manager for a big publishing company who came to see me for a general feeling of worry, depression, and increasing difficulty in getting anything done at work. When I first saw him, he was 53, married with a grown son living out of the house. "Contrary to popular belief among friends, I believe that I peaked in sixth grade," Jack said. "From then on, I had to work hard to keep looking okay, despite the fact that I felt confused and glum."

"I want to do a lot, but I can't seem to grab on to things and make them happen," he continues. "Everybody thinks I'm on top of it. My father, who owned his own successful business, had plans and an agenda for my life, but I couldn't do it. My biggest fear is that people will find out about my limitations. Then they'd rub it in my face and say, 'This is all you really are!'"

Jack was known to his friends as "Mr. Agreeable," always easy going, rich, and successful. "I feel like a pathetic swirl of thoughts when I don't know what's going on. I get confused, anxious, and don't know how to get out of it. I can't bring myself to ask for help. I fake it all day, but have tremendous fear that people will know I'm a failure." Jack had tried several rounds of medications over the years but was generally unsatisfied with the results, and the side effects of low libido were unacceptable to him.

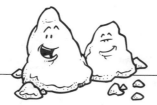

Natural Nuggets

Proper nutrition can be quite helpful in assisting you to cope with anxious feelings. Here are a few tips to get you started:

➤ Avoid caffeine, alcohol, sugar, and refined foods.

➤ Cut back or eliminate foods you may be allergic to (such as dairy products or peanuts).

➤ Eat an abundance of fresh vegetables, whole grains, and protein.

➤ Add calcium (1,000 milligrams daily), magnesium (400 to 600 milligrams daily), and vitamin B complex (50 to 100 milligrams daily) to your daily diet. They can minimize the effects of stress on the nervous system.

In 1980, Jack's life changed when he was awarded a large settlement for an automobile accident he was involved in. "I got into gambling. I was running wild with the excitement and the attention. I could finally be what everyone expected. It's very important for me to have respect and feel important. Then I lost all the money. I tried to hide it from my wife and our friends, but eventually I think they all knew something was wrong."

Jack got into Gambler's Anonymous and became active in his church. "In church, I'm turned to for advice. I like that. I feel like I always have a place at the table." Inside, however, Jack continued to be tortured by the feelings of being a fraud and a failure that haunted him everyday. I prescribed Veratrum Album 12c to be taken daily at a different time of day than his conventional medication.

Over the next few months, Jack noticed he was becoming more functional. "I am more uniformly alert, have good general energy, am less hyper, and not as fussy. I blew a couple of things at work, took the criticism, and didn't try to cover it up. We had a dinner party, and I was more relaxed around people. I'm usually envious of other people's good fortunes, but I was okay."

After six months, he said, "I feel like I've turned over a new leaf. I'm working with my doctor to cut back on my meds in another couple of weeks. I am feeling that I have issues around pride, and have talked to my wife about going in for counseling. I don't get mad now." Jack continued to improve, needing one dose of Veratrum Album 1M after he was off all his medications. He has been off all medications and has not felt the need to take any homeopathics for over a year.

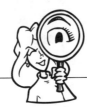

Curious Clues

Veratrum Album is a plant that grows on high elevations in the mountains. People who resonate with this remedy often like the feeling of being above others. Other signs that point to the use of this remedy include ...

➤ Jealousy and envy of others.

➤ Confusion over basic morals of right and wrong.

➤ Feelings of being a great person.

➤ Overly religious, to give outward appearance of being moral.

➤ Overly critical of others, rude.

➤ Loss of social status.

➤ Deceit and lying to show better status.

Panic Attacks: Danger, Danger!

You're in the middle of your day, doing ordinary activities when suddenly your heart begins to pound, sweat begins to pour out of you, and you start to tremble and breathe rapidly. You may be one of the three to six million Americans who suffer from *panic attacks.* During these sudden episodes of uncontrolled terror, many people feel as if they're having a heart attack, going crazy, or even dying. It's a serious medical condition that affects twice as many women as men, often beginning in young adulthood between the ages of 15 and 25. Typically attacks last a couple of terrifying minutes, but they can also be unexplainably prolonged and in rare cases can last one hour or more!

According to the *Merck Manual,* symptoms of panic attacks include ...

➤ Heart palpitations.

➤ Sweating.

➤ Shaking.

➤ Fear of dying.

➤ Fear of going crazy.

➤ Feelings of unreality, strangeness, or being detached from your environment.

➤ Flushes or chills.

➤ Nausea.

➤ Shortness of breath, feeling short-winded.

➤ Trembling or shaking.

➤ Numbness or tingling.

Treatment typically involves medications such as a variety of benzodiazepines like Alprazolam or Clonazepam for anxiety. Supportive psychotherapy and individual, family, or group therapy are also used for long-standing disorders.

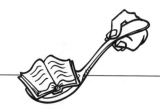

Dose of Info

According to *A Dictionary of Word Origins,* many people with repeated **panic attacks** develop a panic disorder known as agoraphobia, the fear of leaving home or being in a public place. They severely restrict their activities to avoid setting off another attack, until there's no place left to go, but stay home. It affects 3.8 percent of women and 1.8 percent of men. Onset is usually in the early 20s.

Panic Attacks

Larry had his lips pressed tightly together and his arms pinned to his side as he walked to my front desk to ask in a quiet, trembling voice if he was in the right office. A warm greeting did not thaw out the icy exterior of this 19-year-old young man who had come with his mother for help with anxiety and panic attacks. When I asked how long he had been concerned about this condition, he said, "It's been forever. I've been sick from any kind of change all my life." He said that his stomach ached, he felt nauseous, and had sweaty palms. "I feel trapped. I have to make sure wherever I go that I know where all the doors and exits are."

When asked of her pregnancy with Larry, his mother replied, "It was nine months of tension. I was threatened by a miscarriage the entire pregnancy, and was worried all the time about anything and everything. I was just trying to do the right thing." She carried full term and had an uneventful delivery. As an infant, Larry was healthy and met all his developmental milestones. "As a toddler, he couldn't stand the least change in his routine." She thought that might be normal for all toddlers, until a couple of years later he began to turn down any invitation to someone else's home or overnights with the neighborhood kids. "It took us a while to catch on," his mother said, "but when he was invited anywhere, he'd do something awful at home until he got grounded!"

Dose of Info

According to the *Merck Manual*, **habituation** is a form of behavioral therapy that is used in treating phobias, such as agoraphobia, when patients confront their fears. With the support of clinicians and therapists, patients remain in contact with their fears until the anxiety is gradually relieved.

As he grew older, when his environment was not under complete control, he'd get angry. Grade school proved to be a big challenge for Larry. If he couldn't get the answer right the first time, he didn't want to do his schoolwork. His parents became even more worried when he entered high school. "He was sick every morning before high school," his mother recounted. "He never ate breakfast, and I'd have to stop the car on the way to school so he could vomit along the side of the road." His parents took him to their doctor who prescribed Zoloft (an antidepressant similar to Prozac) and antacids. His stomach calmed down somewhat, but he began to develop insomnia and woke up unrefreshed from sleep. His parents were becoming very concerned, especially when he told them he wanted to go to college like everyone else. They did not want to force him to face his fears through *habituation* therapy; instead they were looking for something to bring him out of his protective cocoon.

His first year at college showed a worsening of his condition. "I was obsessed with being perfect," Larry said. "I was an accounting major, because I liked the order and structure. I always wanted to be right and be the best. I superprepared all the time. If I couldn't be the best, or even thought I couldn't be the best, I wouldn't even try. I'd put off the homework or doing a paper until the last minute. Then I would pull an all-nighter to get it done. I'd need to study, but my friends would come over with pizza and want to listen to music and hang out. I couldn't say no." Larry would make himself sick over schoolwork and keep procrastinating, so the stress of college escalated.

During a few minutes of private conversation with his mother, she shared that Larry had kept the same job as a grocery store bagger for the past six years. He'd been asked to do other jobs in the store, even management, but turned them all down saying that he was "comfortable" doing what he had always done. He plays the piano to relieve stress and has had a very awkward time with dating and had no girlfriend for quite some time.

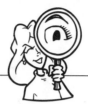

Curious Clues

What would you pick out as the most important imbalances of Larry's story? What homeopathic remedy or family of remedies would be most appropriate to help him? I chose Vanadium, a metal that was discovered in 1830 and is used to increase the hardness of other metals so they don't bend easily, such as in making tools and keys. Here are the points of Larry's condition that I matched up with symptoms associated with Vanadium using Jan Scholten's *Homeopathy and the Elements* (Scholten, 1996):

➤ Tortured by the idea that they might fail

➤ Perfectionism with tasks

➤ Control

➤ Routine, order, and rules

➤ Procrastinating or postponing tasks they may fail at

➤ Suffering from their perfectionism

➤ Overpreparation due to fear of failure

Patients who may benefit from using homeopathic Vanadium generally have fears of failure, criticism, being observed, and being late. Their moods alternate between happy with success and gloomy with failure. They are generally soft and yielding, easily influenced by others, and feel better when under strong control or supervision.

I gave Larry Vanadium 30c and set up a follow-up appointment. One month later, he came in just before his office visit, smiling, and without his mother. "I'm a lot better," he said, "more at ease. I might get nervous one or two times a week instead of from morning till night. The anxiety is shorter in duration and easier to handle. Before,

I couldn't get it out of my head, but now I can." His sleep was more restful, he felt less nauseous, and he fought less with his sisters. He still procrastinated, though. "I have it in my mind to do it, but something just happens."

I advised him to continue the Vanadium, one dose per week, while his mother worked with his doctor to reduce—and finally eliminate—his medications. Over the next two years Larry was seen every three to four months. During that time he became more engaging and responsive, started dating successfully, and stopped procrastinating. He was able to change his major—an important milestone for him—and continues to do well.

Dose of Info

Night terrors are sudden awakening with inconsolable panic and screaming. They usually occur in the first one to three hours of sleep. On waking, the person typically looks confused for a while. They occur most commonly in children age three to eight and are frequently triggered by stressful events.

Night Terrors

Lauren would wake up most nights screaming at the top of her lungs in absolute terror, sure that a shadowy figure stood above her as she slept. She had suffered from insomnia and sleep disturbance most of her life, but the *night terrors* increased when she went to college. "I absolutely believe that someone is standing over my head and is about to harm me and I'm in danger." Sometimes she would skip a few nights, then wake up screaming three or four nights in a row. As a young girl she was never invited to sleepovers, and in college her roommates were understanding, but eventually had to leave. She had occasional menstrual cramps, PMS, tension headaches, and asthma. Otherwise, she felt good as a healthy 19-year old. She grew up in a very close household, and didn't make friends easily. When she did get a date her parents usually did not like him unless he was from the same orthodox religion as she was. "I'm still angry about it, but don't know what to do about it."

Her mother told me that when she was nine months pregnant she found out about a terrible thing her husband had done. She wouldn't talk about it, only saying, "It forever changed what I wanted out of my marriage." Several members of the family knew about this occurrence, but none were allowed to discuss it. "I couldn't even go into labor, I had to be induced, it still upsets me." I gave Lauren Lac Dolphinum 200c, the homeopathic form of dolphin milk.

We met for a follow-up visit in six weeks. "I've been starting to have dreams when I get mad at people who have mistreated me. The night terrors are better, less frequent, but I still have them. Now I wake up startled, but not screaming."

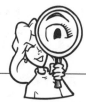

Curious Clues

The homeopathic community uses the experiences of provers (discussed in Chapter 4, "Provings—The Proof Is in the Person") as a basis for our knowledge of Lac Dolphinum. The following are key themes that were also part of Lauren's story:

➤ Family secrets, shameful events

➤ Covering up the truth, hiding

➤ Suppressed anger, which comes out in dreams

➤ Feeling of impending danger

➤ Poor sleep

➤ Disturbing dreams, fitful sleep

Source: Nancy Herick

After five months the night terrors had ceased, she had gotten angry about old abusive boyfriends, and was setting boundaries with her parents and new boyfriends. She was interviewing for a new job. No menstrual cramps or PMS, and her asthma was almost completely resolved. Within another three months, her conditions resolved satisfactorily. Our last visit was for another condition three years later and she told me she still had no night terrors.

Manic Depression: A Season of Emotions

Imagine if the gas pedal of your car would get stuck by itself, going either too fast or too slow. It would be frustrating and disappointing trying to get where you wanted to go when you never know if you'll be in control enough to function. This is what someone who is dealing with manic depression (or bipolar disorder) has to deal with. Depression in some form affects an average of 20 percent of women, 10 percent of men, and 5 percent of adolescents worldwide. An estimated 17.6 million Americans are diagnosed with a major depression every year, while manic depression affects up to three million people in the United States yearly.

The observable symptoms of manic depression show a shift between mania and depression. The mood change is usually inappropriate for the situation.

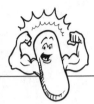

Potent Pellets

An estimated three million Americans suffer from bipolar mental disorder. This can manifest in three distinct ways that are important to recognize:

➤ Bipolar I: manic or high spirits with or without depression

➤ Bipolar II: severe depression and early mild mania

➤ Rapid cycling: frequent alternations of mood extremes

Symptoms of Both States of Manic Depression

Manic Phase

Elevated mood

Agitation

Increased activity

More talkative

Racing thoughts

Restlessness

Inflated self-esteem

Poor temper control

Decreased need for sleep

Increased goal setting or sexual activity

Depressive Phase

Loss of self-esteem

Overwhelming sluggishness

Withdrawal

Daytime sleepiness

Feelings of helplessness, worthlessness

Insomnia

Excessive guilt

Loss of appetite/weight loss

Source: Merck Manual

Treatment may include hospitalization in acute phases, and antidepressants and benzodiazepines are commonly prescribed. Lithium carbonate may be prescribed for maintenance; however, common chronic adverse effects of Lithium include exacerbation of acne, mild psoriasis, hypothyroidism, and nephrogenic diabetes insipidus.

Manic Depression (Presented by Savitri Clarke)

Betty is a 41-year-old woman who enters the consultation room agitated, nervous, and looking suspicious. She begins by telling me how, as a small child, she was full of joy, laughed a lot, and had a bright disposition. From infancy to age seven, she was severely physically and sexually abused by her father. "That left an anger in me that turned into a poison so that I forgot about the abuse in order to survive and then it started to resurface when I was 24."

At 29, she came down with juvenile diabetes. The following year she was diagnosed with depression after going on insulin to try to manage her sugar levels. With the onset of depression she became suicidal and went into a hospital, afraid she would hurt herself. Her mother was also manic-depressive.

"Before the diabetes and depression I was living a healthy lifestyle, lost 15 pounds, exercised, swam, and was in good shape. After this happened, I felt I was already doing everything I knew to heal myself so I embraced Buddhism and started chanting." This seemed to help, but the next year she was depressed again. She went into day treatment and took a leave from work. "It became hard to chant when I was really depressed—because I didn't want to do anything—so I went on antidepressant medication."

Over the next few years, Betty cycled in and out of depression as she began law school. At the end of the first year of law school she started to become manic. "You think you are doing fine. I was having a great time, but becoming more isolated."

"I became paranoid, felt assassins were following me, wouldn't sit near windows. I thought a friend who cooked me dinner was trying to poison me. It was about being

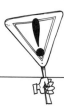

Caution Keeper

According to an article in *Psychosomatic Medicine*, a research study done by the U.S. Centers for Disease Control and Precaution found that depression in white men raised their risk of stroke by 68 percent and in white women by 52 percent, while black men and women were at an astounding 160 percent increased risk of stroke with depression.

Source: July/August 2000 issue of Psychosomatic Medicine

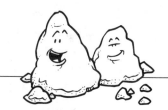

Natural Nuggets

According to researchers at Duke University's Medical Center, exercise may reduce major depressive disorder (MDD) in the long term and may be at least as effective as sertraline (Zoloft). Participants who continued to exercise after the study were even less likely to be classified as depressed.

victimized." Finally Betty was hospitalized, diagnosed with manic depression, put in restraints, and given Haldol. When she came out of the hospital, the "high" was over and she was severely depressed. She was again put on antidepressant medication.

Since law school, Betty works advocating for children who the state suspects are being abused. "I just have so much rage about what happened to me. I think about it all the time."

"Every day I try to manage an unbelievable ocean of emotions. I do it by drinking caffeine, smoking cigarettes, and self-injury by scratching myself." At this point, Betty shows her forearm covered with nickel-size white scars.

"I love sugar, it numbs my feelings. I have to eat a pint of ice cream every night. I know it isn't good for my diabetes but I can't seem to stop myself. I hate myself. I think I am the most disgusting thing. I put on music that is good for me. My sexual energy is very high. I move fast, always hurried, impatient." Betty was given the remedy Tarentula Hispanica, the homeopathic form of the Spanish tarantula spider.

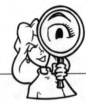

Curious Clues

Betty was given the remedy Tarentula Hispanica, the homeopathic form of the Spanish tarantula spider. People who need animal remedies tend to be intense and have issues of survival, competition, and attracting others. For Betty, the remedy was chosen based on the following symptoms:

➤ Self-torture, scratching or striking herself with rage

➤ Desire for dancing

➤ Better from music (especially music with a strong beat, like chanting, drumming)

➤ High sexual energy

➤ Hurried

➤ Fear of spiders

➤ Changeable mood

➤ Sadness on waking

➤ Diabetes mellitus (Tarentula is a major remedy)

After three years of homeopathic treatment, Betty no longer cycles through depressive and manic phases and is off all medications, except a small amount of antidepressants. During this period, she has entered into a healthy intimate relationship and wants to get married and have a child. She rarely injures herself, is able to work, and her blood sugar has come down. "I feel more empowered towards my healing. I am doing informal research about my diabetes and feeling more like I want to heal it. I would love to be a child psychologist for abused children."

Has Grief Got You Down?

Most of us have experienced a loss at some time in our lives. Whether it's a death of a family pet, loss of a job, financial decline, or being separated from a loved one by death or divorce. Different cultures, genders, ages, and religious beliefs may determine how we initially react to grief.

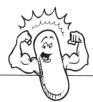

Potent Pellets

According to the Web site www.onhealth.com (see Appendix B), symptoms of general grief may mimic those of depression. Many experts believe that we go through phases during our healing from grief:

➤ Shock: You may feel numb or experience a sense of disbelief. Tears and angry outbursts are common.

➤ Pain: Shock declines, while sadness, loneliness, and depression increase. Fatigue, anxiety, guilt, and restlessness occur.

➤ Healing, reorganization, and integration: Sadness and disbelief may persist, although you gradually develop several interests in work, home, and life.

Health professionals call "complicated grief reaction" a particularly severe form of grieving that lasts an unusually long time. Symptoms of complicated grief response may include ...

➤ Inability to work or impaired function.

➤ Guilt about things done or not done at the time of a loved one's death.

➤ Extreme feelings of worthlessness.

➤ Sleep problems persisting for four to six weeks.

➤ Weight loss exceeding 10 pounds.

➤ Thoughts of death.

➤ Hallucinations.

Treatment is based on the individual's reactions. Time, medication, and counseling may be used depending on the severity of the reaction and the length of time it takes to feel better.

Grief Relief (Presented by Pamela J. Herring)

Bertha's husband was terminally ill with colon cancer, and she was distraught—not because of her fear of losing him, but rather she was angry, unhappy. "He's been a workaholic," she complained. "I feel so empty after all these years of marriage."

When Bertha came in, she appeared very anxious and said she was experiencing a pressure in her chest that extended up to the right side of her neck causing an uncomfortable lump in her throat. She had seen her medical doctor the previous week, but he couldn't find any problem with her heart or anything else, and so dismissed her. Yet she expressed a fear of having a stroke or heart attack. "I have a history of migraines due to anger," she stated. "My husband gave me no help at all. I think he's afraid of me. We just can't seem to communicate." She wept as she told her story, and sighed as she described her keen disappointment about not having the kind of loving relationship she wanted with her husband. Now here she was, being called upon to care for him in his last days.

Bertha was a sturdy 66-year-old woman. She had been a nurse professionally (now retired), and she and her husband had raised three children during their 40-year marriage. She stated, "I'm retired and I'm depressed. My husband has been very sick. I feel trapped. There is a lot required to take care of him these days."

This is a clear case of Ignatia, one of the premier grief remedies and one of the main remedies for "hysteria." In fact, the condition of the lump in the throat is classic. It is often termed "globus hystericus," a ball in the throat caused by an emotional upset. It is always a good idea to rule out heart problems with chest pain, and since this had already been done by her medical doctor before she came in, we could proceed with treating her by giving the indicated remedy for the whole person. Pain in the heart area often accompanies grief. Bertha was given a single dose of Ignatia 200c.

Looking at the nature of Ignatia, it is often indicated where a person has invested his entire emotional life in one person, like a spouse or a child. The Ignatia person (usually a woman, though sometimes useful for men) enjoys being seen as the ideal caretaker, self-sacrificing at her own expense. The one whose love and attention she is seeking may ignore her or is rude to her, and because she is so sensitive, it is heartbreaking to her. The Ignatia woman can become bitter and angry or hysterically upset so that she cannot eat, sleep, or function in her disappointment. The Ignatia woman will also try to suppress her feelings, suffering silently, and doing her duty until, finally, she breaks down from the grief or sadness. She will often break down into sobbing as a desperate attempt to get the attention of the person in whom she is invested emotionally.

Key rubrics of Ignatia from the mind section of the repertory that fit this case include ...

➤ Ailments from grief.

➤ Ailments from anger, vexation with anxiety.

➤ Ailments from anger, vexation with silent grief.

➤ Ailments from disappointment.

➤ Delusions, neglecting her duty (feeling that there are responsibilities left undone).

➤ Ailments from cares.

➤ Moods, changeable.

➤ Cheerfulness followed by melancholy.

➤ Sensitive to rudeness.

On Bertha's return visit one month later, the lump in her throat had completely disappeared, as had her chest pain. She said she had read a book on relationships that had helped. She could finally be at peace with her husband and no longer feel resentment toward him.

Over the next two years, as her husband was dying, Bertha received periodic doses of Ignatia and for about two years afterward, during her adjustment to living without her husband. She was grieved and missed him, often expressing how grateful she was to be able to love him during his dying process. Ignatia helped her to maintain her equilibrium throughout those six years.

As you have seen from the cases in this chapter, a diagnosis of a mental condition can be treated effectively using the principles of homeopathy along with other medical and social support systems. In the next chapter, we'll continue to look at emotions that may not have a diagnosis, yet still create an unbalanced emotional life for us.

The Least You Need to Know

➤ Homeopathic remedies are effective in treating many of the most limiting mental conditions.

➤ Generalized anxiety disorder (GAD) affects 3 to 5 percent of the U.S. population and may run in families.

➤ Adding calcium, magnesium, and vitamin B complex to your daily diet can minimize the effects of GAD.

➤ Panic attacks are twice as likely in women than men, often beginning between ages 15 and 25.

➤ Exercise can minimize the effects of depression as effectively as sertraline (Zoloft).

➤ Complicated grief reaction refers to a severe or long-lasting grieving, characterized by guilt, impaired function, and feeling of worthlessness.

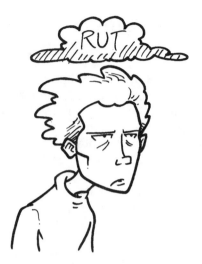

Chapter 10

Getting Stuck in Our Emotions

> ### In This Chapter
>
> ➤ Put stress to rest with homeopathic treatment
>
> ➤ Learn to lose the worry habit the remedy way
>
> ➤ Discover the homeopathic hope available for rampaging rage
>
> ➤ When too much excitement leads to trouble

Have you ever been in a maze? I mean a real hedgerow or corn maze? I was in one recently, and it took me almost 1½ hours to find my way out. I was thinking the whole time to just relax, trying to do intellectual exercises to outthink the maze, as if being smarter would get me out faster. I went through a gambit of emotions, ranging from bewilderment and embarrassment to anger. I even had visions of sleeping on the bench I kept passing over and over again. It didn't make sense. I knew I was safe, but these feelings crowded in anyway and became tough to shake no matter how much I thought about it.

The emotions that you'll read about in this chapter are maze-like in their ability to defy rational thinking. You can become imprisoned in worry, circle around in stress, while running in rage excitably for the exit. No amount of self-convincing seems to extricate us from these common emotions that have temporarily gotten us turned around. Continue reading and learn the homeopathic keys to a successful exit from your mental mazes.

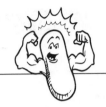

Potent Pellets

Stress can take you down for the count. Its records of knockouts include ...

➤ Seventy-five percent to ninety percent of visits to physicians are stress-related.

➤ Job stress is a major health factor, costing businesses an estimated $150 billion annually.

➤ Fifty percent of all diseases in the United States have a stress-related origin.

➤ Stress-related disorders are a major cause of rapidly increasing health-care costs.

Source: National Mental Health Association

Stress: Guessin' Who's Stressin'

"Hurry up, they've been waiting 45 minutes for you! Why are you so late?" Ugh, this is the bad kind of stress, complete with quickened pulse rate and breathing, a rise in blood pressure, tense muscles, and oh, yes, perspiration. Your body automatically reacts to the "fight-or-flight" scenario in both physical and emotional ways. Some stresses get us motivated or entertain us—like a video game or paint ball. These are usually short-term imposed stresses. When stress overstays welcome, that's when we become noticeably affected.

Do you wake up in neutral each morning, or are you still in gear from the day before? Are you in low gear prepared for tough going as you climb up a steep embankment, in high gear racing by all the rest, or have you put it in reverse heading for the hills?

If you can't get back to neutral with a good night's sleep, then you run the risk of building up increasing amounts of residual stress that you carry around each day. It may even become difficult for you to know that stress is getting to you. Here's a little checklist. If you recognize these as personal characteristics, then you've got stress.

Your Stress Test

(Answering Yes Means You Have Stress)

Yes	No	
❏	❏	Do minor problems and disappointment upset you easily and excessively?
❏	❏	Do the small pleasures of life fail to satisfy you?
❏	❏	Are you unable to stop thinking of your worries?
❏	❏	Are you constantly tired?
❏	❏	Do you experience flashes of anger over situations that used to not bother you?
❏	❏	Have you noticed a change in your sleeping or eating patterns?
❏	❏	Do you feel inadequate or suffer self-doubt?

Source: National Mental Health Association

Knowing your limits is helpful in deciding how much stress to take on. We all handle it differently. Be sure to keep it in check, or you'll be the one checking out!

Stress and Tendinitis (Presented by Savitri Clarke)

Terry came for help with tendinitis in both her arms. She was a soft, sensitive, 30-year-old woman who seemed quite fragile. I saw her holding back tears from the very beginning. She started by saying that the pain in her arms coincided with her husband's long battle with cancer. Both her pain and her husband's health problems got worse a year ago. He is well now, but went through many rounds of unsuccessful chemotherapy before finding something that worked. "I know it was very stressful. A lot of the stress was from having to hold emotions in because I had to perform." My body finally said I couldn't do this anymore."

When her arm pain started to increase, Terry was taking care of her husband at home. After clearly holding it back for a time, she finally started to cry when she said, "I was really scared, scared I was going to lose him. I didn't know for a while during that time if I was helping him live or helping him die. I was afraid I was losing everything."

Now that her husband is doing better, Terry expressed surprise that her symptoms haven't gone away. "I am still dealing with so much; so many of my symptoms haven't gone away."

When asked what would make her pain worse, she said, "It wouldn't have to be a bad stress for my arm pain to get worse. It could be that I would have to speak up about something ... such as a need not being met. I would start burning up in the forearm muscles. It has moved up my arm and now I am tight as a rock in the back of my upper arms and shoulders." She has always had a problem speaking up, worrying about how it will make the other person feel, or how it will look. "I was this sweet child with five adopted siblings, two from India. I was the easy one. My sister who was a year older cried all the time." There wasn't room for Terry to speak up. Her father was unavailable. When her mother visited during her husband's illness Terry was very disappointed. "In my whole life my mother was never able to focus on me. There was always another child in crisis. There has never been room for me. I have never been the crisis child. This was my one moment and she still couldn't be there for me."

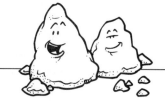

Natural Nuggets

Here is a list of stress-busters to keep in mind:

➤ Get adequate rest, relaxation, and sleep.

➤ Eat a well-balanced diet.

➤ Drink plenty of water.

➤ Drink alcohol only in moderation.

➤ Stay at a healthy weight.

➤ Balance each day between work and personal time.

➤ Exercise three to four days a week for 30 minutes each day.

Source: Debora J. Orick, February 1999, www.drkoop.com

Terry's job as a pianist requires her to play the piano intensely each weekend. She did not have many distinguishing characteristics of her arm pain but it was significant that she could feel the pain increase immediately with stress and performance anxiety. It was clear that the remedy that fit what she had been feeling during this difficult time should also help her tendinitis. She was given the homeopathic remedy Natrum Muriaticum, which is homeopathic sodium chloride (salt).

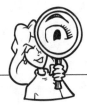

Curious Clues

People who need the remedy Natrum Muriaticum are sensitive, easily hurt, and have a strong need for a relationship. This makes them especially sensitive to disappointment and rejection. They tend to internalize their emotions, to be devoted care givers, and are very reluctant to ask others for help, which they view as burdening others. Their sensitivity to rejection and embarrassment can make public performing quite stressful. They often suffer from feelings of intense sadness and grief.

Terry came back a month later saying, "This is still magic to me! I went home to visit my mother three days after taking the remedy. Our time was tightly packed and there were a lot of things that could draw me in and I could lose my balance easily. But I maintained myself that whole time. I wanted to spend time with my mom. I could just be with her, where she was at, didn't feel frustrated and irritated inside. I was also able to speak my truth with my older sister and we had some bonding times. It was time for me as the younger sister to say 'I need you to get to know me in this way and I want to allow you to get to know me also.' I did that with my dad, too. It was a huge trip for me."

"My arms have improved. I did some physical work that inflamed all of my symptoms, but a few days later I was not feeling the pain. I rebounded much faster than I expected."

Terry was clearly better both emotionally and physically and continued to improve with only occasional doses of her remedy.

Worry: The Brain Drain

Sometimes thoughts keep crowding in like downtown subway riders during rush hour. Just when you think your brain can't create another worrisome creation, you manufacture a *worry* that just manages to squeeze into your mind.

Samuel Hahnemann recognized the potential for illness from prolonged emotions when he wrote in paragraph 225 of *The Organon,* "There are certainly a few emotional diseases that have not simply degenerated from disease. It develops outward from the emotional mind due to persistent worry, mortification, vexation, abuse, or repeated exposure to great fear or fright. While initially there is but little infirmity, in time emotional diseases of this kind often ruin the state of health to a high degree" (Hahnemann, 1996).

Worrying impacts the quality of your life. It's more difficult to enjoy your family on the weekends if thoughts of unfinished work or financial pressures compete with your loved ones for attention. Until excessive worry develops into a condition such as anxiety, depression, or high-blood pressure, there are no specific treatments for worry in conventional medicine. Interestingly enough, there is a growing trend in mind-body approaches that may include relaxation exercises and meditation. While these are always helpful, take a look at a homeopathic solution for the wild worries.

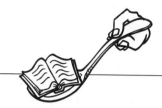

Dose of Info

Worry originally meant "strangle" in prehistoric Germanic (from the word *Wurgjan,* which also produced the word *choke*). The modern sense of "vex" was not commonly used until the mid-nineteenth century. Worry often chokes off the inspirations and strangles our inner wisdom. Learning to let go of worry clears the way for solution thinking to prevail.

Infertility "Worryability" (Presented by Savitri Clarke)

Bob came in with his wife to see if there was anything that would help them in their efforts to have children. They both came from big families and wanted to have 10 children. Unfortunately, it was not as easy as they had expected and they had been trying for two years unsuccessfully. Bob was concerned that his sperm count was low and there was some problem with his morphology (the shape of the sperm). But after we spoke for a while, it was clear that there was another problem Bob wanted help with. He was a constant worrier.

"I worry about work, think about things pending at work. I can get very nervous for other people. If my wife is anxious I can even shake! I worry and get very upset if I think she is upset. I worry about other people being safe. I worry about the future, about our ability to have children, about my family."

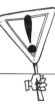

Caution Keeper

Worrisome stresses can evolve to more serious ailments. The list includes such unwelcome conditions such as hypertension, migraine headaches, ulcers, anxiety, allergies, asthma, as well as cancer and cardiovascular disease. These stresses can even make you more susceptible to colds and tooth decay!

Source: drkoop.com

Bob knew that this tendency to worry made him less effective at both his job and home. "I would like to be able to relax more and worry less."

"Things that make me happy are family. Family is very important to me. My job is also very important because I take my role as provider very seriously. That is how I was raised. That is what the man is supposed to do. I am a very sensitive, emotional person and I tend to keep things in."

Bob came from a family of six children. He was the first boy after four girls and his parents describe his birth as "the second coming of Christ!" Bob's parents had high expectations of him as a child. "I tend to be a perfectionist both at work and at home. I can't stand it when things are out of place, dirty, or messy. When I hear bad news or get really nervous, I feel a burning through my veins."

Bob's worry has escalated since dealing with infertility. "I obsess about having a child. If I hear that someone else has had a child, I think about it at work. I have some resentment that other people have children so easily. We are very religious and pray a lot. At times, I want to change religions but I know that is not the answer."

Bob feels he is a failure because they can't have kids. It bothers him that he can't do anything about it. He has a fear of failure and of letting other people down.

Bob also has seasonal allergies with watery, crusty eyes in the morning, itchy eyes and throat, and nasal congestion. He has had some problems with loose stool from nerves or stress. I prescribed Kali Arsenicosum.

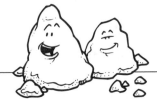

Natural Nuggets

The way you relax is a personal choice. List the top three options that sound good to you and sign up for classes to experience them firsthand. Here are a few options to get you started:

➤ Meditation

➤ Progressive muscle relaxation

➤ Stretching

➤ Deep breathing

➤ Aerobic exercise

➤ Tai chi

➤ Yoga

➤ Massage

Over the next three years Bob's worrying decreased significantly, he was more able to relax about things, and he and his wife were able to have two children. He was able to put his problems at work in perspective and let things go more easily. He said, "My wife is happy that I don't have to have everything cleaned up right away now and that I don't get so uptight any more."

Rage: Mad at the World

Remember the class bullies in school? They had a reputation for taking it out on others, being a loose cannon, getting what they wanted with their fists. Violence and intimidation were their calling card. There was an air of unpredictability about them. You didn't want to be around them if they got bad news, because they "processed things" a bit differently than most people, usually with physical force.

Today hostility and *rage* are often displayed on our roadways. According to the American Automobile Association (AAA), road rage has overtaken drunk driving as the leading hazard on our nation's highways. We've all experienced being cut off in traffic and reeling back as another driver's contorted face and muffled screams are framed behind the car's window. The one-finger salute is often given as a parting gesture to ensure your day begins pleasantly!

Getting a handle on anger and rage is an essential part of achieving overall happiness. What do you do to break the cycle? No need to get upset, homeopathic help is on the way!

Rage: A Loose Cannon

"I've done it all. Been there, done that," said Lenny, who came to my office for relief of chronic headaches and back pain. "I started drinking at age 10. When I was 15, my mother was taken away on Christmas Eve in a straitjacket. She was absolutely insane. My dad was negative. His favorite saying was, 'Don't ever trust anyone.'"

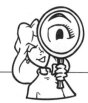

Curious Clues

Bob's sense of duty and conscientiousness about family and his conservative "play by the rules" nature led me to a remedy in the "kali," or potassium, family. His fastidiousness, envy about others having children, constant worrying, religious despair, and sensation of heat in the veins are symptoms of remedies in the arsenic family. I gave Bob the homeopathic remedy Kali Arsenicosum, homeopathic potassium arsenate, also called Fowler's solution.

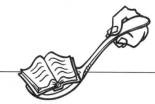

Dose of Info

Rage is a close relative of the word *rabies*. It comes to us via Old French *rage* from the Latin *rabia*, meaning *madness, frenzy, fury*. In French, *rage* still translates as *rabies* as well as *anger*. The intensity of rage is like the fury of a mad dog.

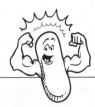

Potent Pellets

A study done by the AAA's Foundation for Traffic Safety shows the following measure of our displeasure behind the wheel:

➤ One out of four road rage incidents occurs between 4 P.M. and 6 P.M.

➤ Sixty-eight percent of road rage occurs on sunny days.

➤ Most incidents happen in the summer (38 percent).

➤ Fridays account for 26 percent of road hostilities.

➤ Holidays and weekends showed no impact in the study.

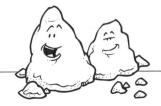

Natural Nuggets

For a quick trip of rest and relaxation, visualize or remember the best vacation you ever took or heard about. Sit quietly with your eyes closed and imagine the sights, sounds, and smells that surround you. Breathe deeply and slowly, enjoying the trip, and at the end of this vacation, there's no tip!

Lenny complained of headaches he had experienced since he was a teenager and low-back pain with sciatica, sometimes in both legs that seemed to get worse when he gets mad. "I always had a terrible temper. In high school a gang member approached me and started to fight me. I pulled out a hammer and beat him! I'd have killed him if they hadn't pulled me off him. They gave me detention for one year. I quit school. Later, my dad kicked me out of the house, so I joined the navy and became an even meaner drunk. I was cruel."

Lenny got out of the Navy, married a woman he hated, and divorced her 15 years later. He stopped drinking after that and joined AA. "There's a terrible struggle that's going on inside of me to find truth and peace, but I'm so negative. I'm screwed."

Lenny stated that he was always dealing with getting crazy. "I have fantasies of running over people and killing them. I've battled negative thinking my whole life. When I get like this, my head pounds and my back tightens up. I can barely walk." I gave Lenny the remedy Lachesis, the homeopathic dilution from the Bushmaster snake.

Over the past three years, Lenny has been able to hold down a good job, has become a sponsor in AA, and interacts with his children and ex-wife in nonviolent ways. He's had bouts of anger, but does not get stuck in them and is able to find solutions to conflict without getting into a shouting match or a fistfight. He's become happier, went to counseling, and has an air of humor and joy about him. His headaches and back pain left fairly soon after the remedy and have not been a significant discomfort despite numerous physical activities. "I'm on more of a spiritual quest than I have ever been."

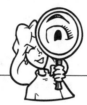

Curious Clues

Did you notice the serpent's signs? Patients who would benefit from the homeopathic remedy of Lachesis display such traits as ...

➤ Passionate, intense.

➤ Talkative or loquatious.

➤ Anger, aggression.

➤ Hatred, rage, longing for revenge.

➤ Chronic headaches.

➤ Depressed and anxious.

➤ Disappointment.

➤ Alcoholism, drug abuse.

➤ Back pain.

➤ Sciatica, one- or two-sided.

Overexcitement and Stimulation

Extreme paragliding, death-defying mountain biking, and unbelievable killer snow-boarding are just a few examples of what I've observed as society's preoccupation with extreme excitement. No longer is it acceptable to be thrilled. Your sports, television, movies, and automobile must transport you to terror, giving you sensations of a "brush with death" then bring you back again. This can trick your body into the old "fight-or-flight" mode, but continued doses of this powerful peril could cancel your return ticket and leave your sympathetic nervous system stranded in overdrive.

Samuel Hahnemann had to deal with conditions that arise out of the emotional state and saw that homeopathics were the best way to treat them. "In cases of mental or emotional disease (which are incredibly various), if the selected remedy for a particular case is entirely appropriate for the truly sketched image of the disease state, then the smallest possible doses are often sufficient to produce the most striking improvement" (O'Reilly, 1996). Keep reading to find out how a common stimulant in our culture can help to heal in the homeopathic form.

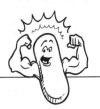

Potent Pellets

The sympathetic nervous system prepares the body for action. When you feel thwarted or excited, your body goes into a series of reactions designed to give you a fighting chance. You get hopping with the help of the adrenal glands that release large quantities of glucose to the liver for an extra source of energy for your muscles. Your heart beats briskly, pupils dilate, and your blood pressure rises, getting you ready to go!

Headaches: Percolating Passions (Presented by Savitri Clarke)

Jill is coming to my office for help with her migraine headaches. She is a vivacious 39-year-old woman who seems quite energized and excited. She makes jokes on the way into my office, and I quickly realize that this is going to be a fun session. She begins talking immediately and we are off to the races!

"My migraines are getting worse. I must be perimenopausal. They are especially bad with ovulation and after my period. The interesting thing about my work is that when I get excited I get a headache. It can be that someone upsets me or I am just happily excited about something and *wham,* a headache!"

As Jill is very open and talks easily, I find out quickly that she is very sensitive to the suffering of others and will always champion the underdog. It is clear that she has a very good heart. Her emotions are right under the surface and can percolate up at any moment. I notice that her face is quite flushed and when I ask about that, she says that it can feel very hot and burning.

"Everyone says I am always so hyper. But I am not so much hyper as interested in things, excited about them, I enjoy what I do. As a child I talked a lot, had a lot of energy, was sarcastic, flip, funny, getting in trouble. I was told to tone down and just sit. I can't do that. Thoughts just keep rushing in. I have to be doing something. I am a fast thinker. I can get easily outraged. I am outspoken. I take risks. I love the outdoors, green is my favorite color." Jill's migraines almost always start on the right side. Certain foods can set them off as can noises and smells, like perfume. "I get very irritable."

I note that Jill is very sensitive physically and emotionally and strongly reactive to her environment. This often indicates a plant remedy.

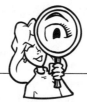

Curious Clues

Individuals who would benefit from the homeopathic remedy Coffea Cruda often display the following symptoms:

➤ Loquacity

➤ Love of the outdoors, nature, the color green

➤ Benevolence

➤ Rapid rush of thoughts

➤ Migraine headache

➤ Headache from excessive joy, after excitement of the emotions, from noise, or after vexation

➤ Extreme irritability is experienced along with pain

➤ Condition is improved with open air

Jill was very creative. It seemed as though she could barely keep up verbally with the thoughts rushing through her mind. As I considered what remedy would help Jill, I realized that she seemed buzzed, like someone would be on too much coffee. I asked her if that was, in fact, the case and she said no she couldn't drink coffee but she did love it. The remedy Coffea Cruda, homeopathic coffee, included all of Jill's symptoms. She was given one dose of the remedy with instructions to stay off coffee for the next month.

When Jill came in for her follow-up appointment one month later, she reported that she had a weird headache the day after the remedy. It was not a migraine and seemed to be related to caffeine withdrawal. Five days after that, she started to get a headache but it began on the left side. Jill did as I had suggested and took another dose of her remedy. Usually her headaches lasted three or four days. This one was gone the next day. She noticed that when she started to get the headache she felt the need to loosen the belt from around her waist. That was a nice confirmation for the remedy Coffea, which gets aggravated from clothing around the waist. She reported, "The next day I felt in a really good mood and more focused. I feel healthier in general." She also reported that she had not had any headaches—even the standard one that always followed her menstrual cycle—since. "I feel more focused, more even, more grounded, calmer."

Over the next nine months, Jill had only a few minor headaches and was able to go back to drinking a moderate amount of coffee.

The conditions we've discussed in this chapter have been more like overwhelming feelings rather than diagnoses. Homeopathic medical philosophy recognizes that when emotions get stuck, symptoms turn to more severe diagnoses. I believe that emotions are best used quickly like fresh fruit. If you try to hold onto them too long, you'll get a mess on your hands.

The next chapter moves into the health of our children. You'll want to keep your "little ones" healthy and happy with homeopathic care.

The Least You Need to Know

➤ Seventy-five percent to ninety percent of visits to physicians are stress-related.

➤ Take the time for rest, relaxation, and sleep to lessen stress.

➤ Excessive worry can lead to anxiety, depression, or high blood pressure.

➤ Control your rage with peaceful images and sense-filled scenes.

➤ Homeopathic forms of coffee can help with headaches, irritability, and rapid thoughts.

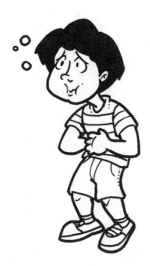

Chapter 11

Childhood Challenges

In This Chapter

➤ Curb colic with homeopathy

➤ End irritating ear infections the homeopathic way

➤ Discover solutions for arresting pediatric asthma

➤ Find out how homeopathy soothes school-time stomachaches

"Mommy, I don't feel good." Don't you have to stop yourself from going into Nurse Mommy mode immediately? It's no better when Daddy's little girl or boy is acting sluggish and unhappy. What's wrong and what can we do?

This chapter will cover some of the most common childhood challenges that parents have to face. While there are a wide variety of pediatric illnesses, both acute and chronic, that homeopathic medicines may effectively treat, I've chosen colic, chronic ear infections, pediatric asthma, and anxious stomachaches as illustrations of how they work.

Homeopathic remedies are safe, nontoxic, and nonhabit-forming health-care options that have become increasingly used by families for the treatment and management of many of today's childhood ailments. I believe that parents will find this chapter particularly helpful in addressing the cycle of illnesses that continually interrupt the happy lives of their children.

Colic: Pass the Gas, Please!

It's easy to feel bad when your baby cries. I've had many new parents sit down looking bedraggled from sleep deprivation, while stacking the blame squarely on their shoulders for an unhappy baby. Rest assured that you are usually not the direct cause of colic, but there are some action steps you can take that may help transform your home into that peaceful abode you've dreamed of.

Colic is common, affecting an estimated 8 percent to 40 percent of infants in their first few weeks of life and disappearing at about three or four months of age. Remember that the official diagnosis of colic is given in threes. If your baby has been crying for more than three hours a day, more than three days a week, and for more than three weeks, he has colic, and you've most likely gone crazy trying to "do something."

The word *colic* pertains to the colon (intestines) and is also called "the gripe" (pronounced grip), because of the feelings we believe your baby is going through with squeezing and grabbing abdominal pain. Typically, colicky infants are healthy, gain weight, and excessive crying has not been shown to be harmful. The difficulty arises from watching your newborn suffer and having your nerves on edge for months at a time.

Breast- and formula-fed babies seem to have the same amount of colic. If you are using a formula, try switching to another brand or a nondairy variety to see if food allergies or intolerances may be contributing to your baby's bothersome belly. Overfeeding is also a common cause of colic, because the infant is often excessively hungry and sucks vigorously on almost anything available. This is a mother's natural cue to feed. While feeding on demand is controversial among child-rearing experts, try scheduled feedings of set amounts of food and observe if colicky symptoms improve.

Homeopathy is frequently used to ease the discomfort of colicky babies. Janice's story below will give you an idea of how combining homeopathic treatment with the suggestions I've just discussed can make a significant change in the quality of babies' and parent's lives.

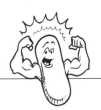

Potent Pellets

Researchers in Denmark have produced a recent study that showed that babies born weighing less than 5.5 pounds were twice as likely to have colic than heavier infants. Other factors that increased a child's likelihood of developing colic were early gestational age, maternal age over 35, and maternal smoking.

Source: Archives of Diseases in Childhood, Fetal and Neonatal, *2000 Edition*

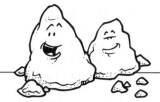

Natural Nuggets

Trapped gas is usually thought of as a source of colic cramping. Breast-feeding mothers may want to avoid eating these gas-producing foods and watch to see if the colic improves.

- ➤ Broccoli
- ➤ Cabbage
- ➤ Cauliflower
- ➤ Brussels sprouts
- ➤ Coffee
- ➤ Rhubarb
- ➤ Garlic

- ➤ Beans
- ➤ Citrus fruits
- ➤ Chocolate
- ➤ Peaches
- ➤ Onions
- ➤ Tomatoes

Source: Prescription for Nutritional Healing

Colic

"She just cries constantly," said Janice's mother when she came to my office for a consultation on treating colic. "She's gassy and uncomfortable; we just don't know what to do." Janice's mother had a normal pregnancy with no complications and Janice was born weighing 7 pounds, 14 ounces, in natural childbirth. "She was always hungry, but was never calm after breast-feeding. She would wiggle around; in fact, she moved a lot when I was pregnant."

Janice began to cry all the time, seemed worse after she ate, and wasn't initially any better with a bowel movement, which usually was runny diarrhea. She was changed from breast-feeding to several different formulas and had tested negative for milk allergies. She was examined by her pediatrician and given the diagnosis of colic. "After feeding, she begins to kick until she's exhausted and falls asleep. She's difficult to hold, because she moves around so much; even sleeping we see her stretching all the time." Janice would usually toss and turn, kicking her covers off. Her mother related that she felt better being held face down and having her back rubbed, but that she seemed still irritable and ill-tempered.

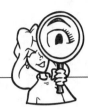

Curious Clues

Have you identified the particular symptoms in Janice's story? They pointed me toward Colocynthis, the homeopathic form of a bitter apple:

➤ Impatient, irritable

➤ Abdominal pain, relieved by pressing on abdomen

➤ Restless with pain

➤ Abdominal pain, relieved by laying face down

➤ Severe cramping pains in the abdomen, with diarrhea

➤ Colic, worse after eating

With a few days of giving Colocynthis, Janice's crying lessened and her overall restlessness decreased. Her parents continued Janice on formula and her colic was gone within a week. Gas decreased and her bowels became more regular and less runny. Janice's parents got sleep and peace of mind, all from a little homeopathic apple.

Ear Infections: Hear Another Way to Save the Day

The desire to ease the pain of *ear infections* drove 30 million parents in America to visit their doctor's office in 1997. This is a three-fold increase in office visits since 1975 for this all-too-common malady. Conventional physicians look for signs of fluid, fever, redness, swelling, and tenderness behind the ear. Acute infections are generally treated with antibiotics, while in chronic infections the ear canal and middle ear are thoroughly cleaned with suction and dry cotton, eardrops, or antibiotics may also be prescribed.

Most ear infections occur when your child is between three months and three years old. This is a time when many new parents are still unsure of what is the right thing to do. This is complicated by the fact that ear infections often happen during the many firsts your child will experience such as the transition from breast milk to formula, the start of solid foods, or the onset of teething. Pressure from anxious parents has long been cited by physicians as the reason antibiotics are so frequently prescribed. Recently there has been more reluctance to overprescribe medications, due to a growing concern of your child developing antibiotic-resistant bacteria. Researchers have found drug-resistant bacteria lurking in the throats of children who had recently had a course of antibiotics.

What's a parent to do? Know that it may take up to three months for the fluid behind your child's eardrum to fully disappear. The existence of fluid is not a sign of impending infections or failed antibiotics. Another medication will just make the fluid in their ears sterile, but will not help it drain. If the fluid takes more than three months to exit, it's time to consider other strategies. Inserting ear tubes to improve drainage is common. As you'll read about next, homeopathic treatment is quickly becoming an effective solution for treating ear infections.

Chronic Ear Infections

Joy's parents must have had a premonition when they chose her name. She was a delightful one-year-old whose engaging smile and infectious giggles had charmed the office staff by the time she came in for her appointment. Her parents were desperate to find a solution for the series of ear infections that Joy had experienced since she attended day care almost six months ago. This was also the time she was switched from breast milk to formula. Joy's mother talked about a smooth, stress-free pregnancy with an uncomplicated delivery. "Joy has always been a happy baby, always smiling, laughing, willing to be held by anyone."

She developed a cold after being in day care, and Joy was taken to her pediatrician who diagnosed her with acute otitis media and prescribed antibiotics. While on the medication, Joy's temperament would change to quiet, fatigued, and jumpy. Her skin was becoming dry, and would get worse when she was hot. Her bowel movements became loose and runny. Her stomach felt better while she drank cold liquids. She normally had a strong appetite, which was also decreased when taking antibiotics. She loved milk, cheese, little wheat crackers, and juice.

Joy was given the homeopathic remedy Phosphorus, a mineral listed on the periodic table of elements. Her parents noticed that over the next few days, her nose became unstuffy and her energy and bright-eyed spirit returned. She felt fine at day care, and on her next pediatric visit her ears still had some fluid, but the redness was gone. The doctor suggested she take a low-dose antibiotic for a year. Her parents took the prescription but never filled it. I also suggested they begin sprinkling probiotic supplements of acidophilus and bifidus into her formula or water. These are naturally occurring healthy bacteria that aid digestion in the intestines and are killed off by antibiotic use. Her parents also began finding alternative foods and gradually, over the course of the next month, eliminated the dairy, sugar, and wheat from her diet.

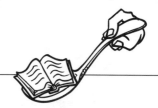

Dose of Info

The American Academy of Pediatrics distinguish between two kinds of **ear infections:**

➤ Acute otitis media—symptoms of ear pain, fever, and pus behind the eardrum. Antibiotics are usually prescribed for this condition.

➤ Otitis media with effusion—fluid in the middle ear. There may also be a temporary loss of hearing, which will return after the fluid drains. Cleaning, monitoring the fluid, ear tubes, or antibiotics are frequently recommended.

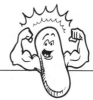

Potent Pellets

Studies show acute otitis media (ear infection), characterized by fever, pain, and pus, resolves within 14 days in 80 percent of children without any treatment. Using antibiotics raises the percentage only to 95.

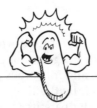

Potent Pellets

Homeopathic treatment of acute otitis media has recently been compared with conventional therapy by the International Clinicians of Pharmacological Therapies. The study involved 103 children in group A (using homeopathic remedies) and 28 children in group B (receiving nasal drops, antibiotics, secnetolytics, and/or antipyretics). Only 5 of the 103 children in group A eventually received antibiotics, and the remaining 98 children had good outcomes. Of the children in group A, 70.7 percent were still free of recurrence within a year, suggesting that homeopathy should be considered as a first-line therapy for otitis media.

Source: Alternative Therapies, *November 1997*

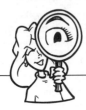

Curious Clues

There are several hints for selecting Phosphorus for Joy's remedy. Did you pick them out?

➤ Open, bright, engaging personality

➤ Stomach feels better after cold liquids

➤ Ear infections

➤ Ravenous appetite; craves milk and cheese

➤ Dry skin, worse from heat

Joy has had several colds since that time and has never developed another ear infection. Her parents use the homeopathic Phosphorous when she gets sick, tired, and anxious; otherwise, they don't give her anything and they report she is her old engaging self again.

Asthma: Begin to Breathe Easy

At almost epidemic proportions, asthma has become one of the most rapidly increasing diseases around the globe. The National Heart, Lung, and Blood Institute (NHLBI) hoped to draw attention to the rapid increase of asthma by marking May 3rd World Asthma Day. Its director, Dr. Claude Lenfant, said, "Although there are still more adults than children suffering from asthma, the increase has been fastest among children and most rapid in preschool-aged children."

In the United States, the number of asthmatics of all ages has more than doubled from 6.7 million in 1980 to an estimated 14.9 million in 1995. The World Health Organization (WHO) estimates that approximately 150 million people around the world suffer from asthma and more than 180,000 die of it every year.

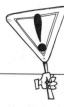

Caution Keeper

Parents who don't let their children get dirty or play with others may be hurting their health. Researchers at The Asthma and Allergy Research Center at the University of Medicine and Dentistry of New Jersey in Newark are suggesting that infants exposed to other children and their germs are less likely to develop asthma later on in life. The first six months is key to exposure of enough germs to stimulate the proper development of their immune systems. Children who attended day care or had two or more older siblings were 50 percent less likely to develop asthma by age 13.

Asthma is a condition that blocks the flow of air into your lungs. During an asthmatic attack, spasms in the muscle surrounding the bronchi (small airways in the lungs) make the air passages smaller, giving you the feeling of sucking your breath through a straw. Coughing, wheezing (the raspy, sucking sound as you breathe), and tightness in your chest are uncomfortable common symptoms of this condition.

Causes for asthma are varied, including viral infections and exposure to allergenic materials such as environmental pollutants, tobacco smoke, chemicals, or fumes. Genetics, exercise, medications, weather changes, stress, and strong emotions have also been noted as triggers for this frustrating and often debilitating condition. Treatment often involves anti-inflammatory medications and quick-relief bronchodilators (inhalers) to treat acute attacks. Many of these medications have significant side effects, and often carry a stigma for children who use them.

Asthma is one of the most disappointing diagnoses for young children to receive, because it often restricts their activities. I'm truly grateful that homeopathic medicines, as you will see, offer effective and safe help for those suffering from asthma.

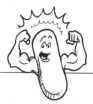

Potent Pellets

Homeopathic medicines have been tested for their effectiveness on patients with corticosteroid–dependent bronchial asthma. The results showed homeopathic therapy led to an improvement in the clinical symptoms compared to a placebo, and allowed for a reduction of the dosage of medications. They concluded that homeopathic treatment appears effective with fewer side effects than standard medications.

Source: Alternative Therapies, *November 1997*

Allergic Asthma

John was a normal 15-year-old boy who wanted to play on the golf and basketball teams and dreamed of summers without itchy eyes, a stuffed-up nose, and irritating asthma. He impressed me as an overly polite young man who exercised an almost military-like rigidity over his upper body while he sat wiggling and bouncing his legs. His mother said she had developed allergies during her pregnancy but otherwise felt fine and had a normal delivery. "John was always a little uptight and anxious about everything, but he was healthy," his mom said. About six years ago, he began to have sinus problems, was diagnosed with allergies, and used medications that seemed to help. He developed pneumonia about two years ago and has been dependent on medications and inhalers ever since. He carried an inhaler everywhere he went; he was afraid that he would forget it, so he obsessed about having it close to him and panicked if he felt like he forgot it.

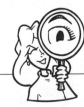

Curious Clues

Arsenicum Album has some distinct signs and symptoms. Have you been keeping track of the particularly individual characteristics of John's asthma?

➤ Anxious, tense, worried

➤ Overly formal, difficult to relax with others

➤ Anxiety about health

➤ Restless and fidgety

➤ Fears that something bad will happen to themselves or their family

➤ Chilly

➤ Burning discharges

➤ Allergies and hay fever

➤ Asthma, worse from midnight to 2 A.M.

John complained about being cold all the time with runny itchy ears, eyes, and nasal discharge. He had most of the common asthma characteristics, including wheezing, which worsened around midnight and with exercise. He was nervous at school, which made it difficult for him to make friends. His mother was concerned that he had developed increasing fears of other illnesses he might catch or problems in the family or burglary, death, or disease. I gave John Arsenicum Album, the diluted homeopathic form of arsenic.

When he first looked at it, he said, "What are you trying to do, kill me?" I explained that the substance he was about to take had no molecules of arsenic left in it, and that it had been carefully prepared in order to be safe to use. In six weeks, John reported the episodes of asthmatic attacks had been cut in frequency and intensity. Sneezing fits were reduced, and he was trying out for the basketball team. In another six weeks, the use of his inhaler had dramatically decreased, especially with exercise and at night. His mother thought he was less nervous and seemed more comfortable inside himself. "His teachers said he was easygoing; that's a new one!" I saw John about every six months for a couple of years. He no longer used his inhaler and finally stopped carrying it around. I saw him three years later at a community event. He said he was happy and never even thought about allergies or asthma.

Stomachaches

"Mommy, my stomach hurts; I don't think I can go to school." Remember hearing this? Remember saying it when that awful test or special project was due when you were in school? The plea from our wee ones to spare them the gauntlet of classroom guidance can be overwhelming.

I've included this condition in this chapter because I've found homeopathic treatments to be both effective and safe, while averting potential personality changes that could shape your child's view of himself in the future.

Anxious Stomachache

"I hate school. I have a teacher who yells. I have never liked school." Twelve-year-old Shelly would come out of her mild moods to periodically rail quietly against school. She sat as far away from her mother and I as possible, with half of her body hidden behind my exam table. Her voice is faint and it is difficult to understand the quiet breathy whispers that she utters after endlessly looking at her mother with expectations that she would do all the talking. Her mother tells me she has a stomachache almost everyday before school and has been that way for years. Complete with nausea, occasional vomiting, severe hiccups, and a full feeling in her stomach. She doesn't want to eat breakfast and complains of pain and pressure in her stomach.

In third grade, she also developed itchy red eczema on her hands. In the fourth grade, she would worry about bad grades, even though she never had any. Shelly followed by whispering, "When the teacher yells at the class, I feel like she's singling me out." "She's a middle child," her mother said. "Her sisters used to bug her, and their grandmother use to live with us and yell at them all the time. She takes everything so personally." I gave Shelly the diluted homeopathic mineral Baryta Carbonicum.

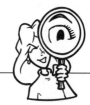

Curious Clues

What did you pick out of Shelly's story that would point you toward a remedy? Baryta Carbonicum is characterized by ...

➤ Being bashful and timid.

➤ Feelings of being watched or laughed at.

➤ Fears of being incompetent.

➤ Desires reassurance.

➤ Feels secure at home, refuses to leave.

➤ School phobias.

➤ Eczema; itchy and red.

➤ Stomach pain, fullness, nausea, loss of appetite.

I noticed at our two-month follow-up that Shelly was sitting next to my desk and not far away out of sight. She was more animated. Her mother said she was getting better at "letting go" of anxiety, and that her hands were beginning to clear up. Shelly is still quiet and reserved, but makes good eye contact and is more engaging in the conversation. This evolution continued over the course of the next six months when she had no stomach pains before school, the eczema had cleared up completely, and she was able to smile, laugh at her mom's jokes, join in school events, and worry less about what others thought of her. I saw her a year later for another condition, and she was doing great. Both Shelly and her mother were relieved to make a break from the stomachache!

Homeopathic treatments are changing the way we think about options for illnesses. As more studies are done and more families successfully use these nontoxic approaches, integration into our health-care system may be possible, as it has been in other countries.

In the next chapter, we will continue with the childhood conditions that can be very challenging: attention deficit disorder, obsessive-compulsive disorder, and bed-wetting.

The Least You Need to Know

➤ Curb colic with homeopathic remedies and by eliminating gassy foods.

➤ Recent studies show homeopathy is effective treatment for acute otitis media (ear infections).

➤ Choosing homeopathic medicines by the totality of symptoms, even for a child, is the most effective way to halt illnesses and promote health for your child.

➤ Keeping your baby safe from the germs of the outside world during the first six months could prevent proper development of his immune system.

➤ Homeopathic help is available for asthma sufferers.

➤ Give school-time anxiety-induced stomachaches recess with homeopathic remedies.

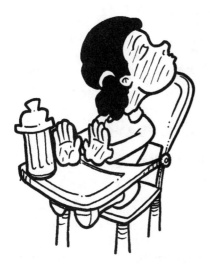

Kid Concerns

In This Chapter

➤ Learn how to deal with picky eaters

➤ Treating obsessive-compulsive disorder

➤ How homeopathy can help with bed-wetting

➤ Attention deficit disorder and homeopathics

Familiar slogans such as "We're winning the war against crime," "Giving your body a fighting chance," or "Battling back to health" suggest that there's a war going on and medicine should choose sides and kick butt! What if the war involves the child you love? Who's the enemy you'll do battle with? Most of the parents I've spoken with whose children struggle with the diagnoses that you'll be reading about would gladly vent their frustrations on a clearly defined foe. The war analogy falls short when you look into the troubled eyes of your child.

You'll be glad to know that homeopathic treatment can move some of these mysterious mountains to aid your family in regaining its balance. The entire family is involved when one of its members is displaying symptoms of attention deficit disorder with hyperactivity, eating disorders, and obsessive-compulsive disorders. The word *disorder* aptly describes the confusion and frustration that often accompanies these conditions.

Bed-wetting affects between five and seven million children each year, but the disappointment and self-imposed stigmas are often kept within the family. This chapter will focus on unlocking your body, mind, and spirit's potential for healing. Let's agree to a cease-fire for our children's sake and examine the benefits of uniting, strengthening, and compassionate care.

Dose of Info

Obsessive-compulsive disorder (OCD) is characterized by recurrent, unwanted, intrusive ideas, images, or impulses that seem silly, weird, nasty, or horrible (obsessions), and by urges to do something that will lessen the discomfort due to the obsessions (compulsions).

Source: Merck Manual, 17th Edition

Obsessive–Compulsive Disorder: Derailing the Rituals

Most of us have little quirks about something we check on that we are uncomfortable with, but with *obsessive-compulsive disorder* (OCD), the behaviors often interfere with everyday routines, jobs, and relationships.

Persons can obsess about anything including contamination, doubt, loss, and aggression. The rituals may logically fit an obsession such as frequently washing your hands for eight hours due to fear of contamination, or may be random as repetitive counting. The condition is chronic, cannot be controlled voluntarily, and may occur without any apparent cause. Since most OCD conditions begin gradually, check with your health-care provider if you notice these symptoms in a loved one.

Symptoms of OCD

For obsession

Involuntary and persistent thoughts that appear to be senseless and cause anxiety or distress

Attempts to suppress the thoughts

Recognition that these thoughts come from one's own imagination, not from outside factors (not always true with children)

For compulsions

Repetitive acts such as hand-washing, checking and rechecking locks, cleaning, repetitive words

Recognition that the behavior is excessive

Depression and distress as attempts to deal with compulsions fail

For children

Ritualistic or compulsive behaviors

Mute behavior with agitated depression

Gradual decline in schoolwork, impaired concentration

Withdrawal and social isolation accompanied by delusional thinking

Mood swings from anxiety to despair

The fear of embarrassment and stigmatization still motivates individuals to conceal this condition. Depression is present in about one third of patients at the time of diagnosis and two thirds during some point in their lives. Treatment combines drug therapy with extensive behavioral therapy that often involves the individual being exposed to the places, faces, or situations that often trigger these attacks. In my experience, homeopathic treatment does not replace any of the behavioral therapies used to help people diminish their discomforts. Using remedies can be an especially useful tool assisting all practitioners to make progress in their patients' care.

OCD Relief

"My daughter is a type A personality who gets stressed over little things. She's a very intense, organized girl who has to have things done a certain way or she'll become overwhelmed and anxious."

Judy was nine years old when her baby sister was born and her parents became concerned about her behavior. "She started washing her hands all the time. It's gotten so bad she now carries her own soap!"

Judy's parents said that over the last two years she's begun repeating phrases incisively, has many rituals at home such as dishes being done a certain way and stacked in the exact order that she dictates. Judy had also developed asthma, which became worse with exercise and anxiety. She has frequent headaches in the back of her head. Her level of anxiety continued to escalate out of control. She was given a diagnosis of obsessive-compulsive disorder by her physician. They tried medication, which only dulled her, so they have gone back to a family-based behavior therapy.

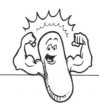

Potent Pellets

In *Lectures on Homeopathic Philosophy*, James Kent discusses how homeopathy delivers an ideal treatment (Kent, 1981):

➤ It restores health and doesn't just remove symptoms.

➤ Treatment must be done promptly, mildly, and establish permanent health.

➤ Use sound, fixed principles of homeopathy, not guesswork, roundabout methods, or cut-and-dried use of drugs as laid down by the last manufacturer. This refers to the latest quick fix being marketed by drug companies.

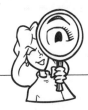

"My work has to be perfect," Judy said. "If I get less than an A, I'm nervous, I cry, and get angry at myself. If I get a homework assignment that's due in a week, I have to do it in a day. I get nervous, can't sleep, and walk around the house at night doing stuff. I want to do well so my family is proud of me."

On our two-month follow-up, Judy's mother said she was generally better and less nervous. She did not need to use her inhaler as much, had not complained of headaches, and was sleeping more often. She still exhibited OCD behavior and perfectionism, but not as consistently.

"Judy's pretty good," her mother exclaimed after four months of homeopathic treatment. "She got a 'C' on a paper and said it was no big deal. She's starting to act like her old self, laughing, joking with the other kids. Her self-blame and anger are much better. She no longer carries around soap. The asthma is greatly improved despite it being the fall, which is her worst time."

During the next six months, she continued decreasing ritual behaviors, helping around the house, but letting go of many of the control issues in her life. She went on a family vacation, had fun, and was able to relax. She got her first "B" on a report card and was okay with it. Her family continued their behavior therapy throughout the course of homeopathic treatment. She continued to improve, getting off all medications, and enjoying school and family life over the next several years. Homeopathy added a valuable component to Judy's efforts to be well.

Diet Dilemmas: Fussy with Foods

"I don't want to eat that, it looks funny." As a parent, you're challenged to figure out what foods are the most nutritious and cost effective for your family. After wading through a rushing stream of often contradictory information, just when you've made peace with your choices, your children veto your vegetable surprise. If we're lucky, it's just a brief phase of finicky eating that frustrates all concerned until a happy medium is found.

Parents do, however, need to be mindful and watch for undue stress around food or body image. Researchers at Stanford University School of Medicine recently interviewed 62 students in grades three through six about their body weight. They found boys and girls were equally dissatisfied with their bodies, and 10 percent had attempted to lose weight. Seventy-seven percent of kids said parents and relatives are their primary source of information about weight loss, while 55 percent cited television and other media sources as important sources. The study appeared in the January issue of the *International Journal of Eating Disorders*.

As I've stated before, homeopathic treatment complements but does not replace good commonsense and skilled behavioral therapists. I hope you will see in Roberto's story that including homeopathic care can make a dramatic contribution to a successful outcome.

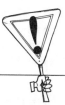

Caution Keeper

Eating disorders may cluster in families. A new study at the University of Pittsburgh suggests that a combination of family genetic influences play an important role in determining susceptibility to eating disorders. The rate of bulimia nervosa and anorexia nervosa among female relatives of persons with eating disorders was between 4 and 11 times higher. Researchers estimate genetic factors contribute 58 percent of risk for eating disorders.

Food Sensitivities (Presented by Savitri Clarke)

Roberto is a charming but soft-spoken and rather shy five-year-old. His mother is getting desperate. Roberto will eat very few foods and his mother is worried his nutritional needs could not possibly be met by his diet. He eats only french fries, pancakes, chips, peanut butter, crackers, and tomatoes. In fact he will eat several tomatoes at a time as if they are apples! He won't try new things.

Roberto has started getting headaches and complains of stomachaches all the time. He gags a lot. "He won't eat at the table with us. He has to have his own little table-cloth and small dish. He won't sit at the table with the cheese still left on the table."

"I start gagging," Roberto says. "I don't want to look at it. I will see the food I don't like and gag. "He went to a party at Chuck E. Cheese's and started to gag when the pizza was set down next to him. He now has a cough and will frequently gag with the cough."

"Sometimes I have stomachaches when I get full."

His mother says, "He doesn't want to finish eating. He says he has a tummy ache and that it hurts around his belly button. My rubbing it makes it better."

Roberto is very good at karate and has no fear. Roberto exclaims, "I am not afraid of anything!"

When I asked about his sleep and dreams, he offered, "I sleep good. Once I dreamt of my head cut off. It was a devil. I was not in bed. I was somewhere else. A place where the devil is, in hell. I was scared.

I asked Roberto about his fears. "I am afraid of monsters, some bugs, spiders, scorpions, snakes, termites. The tail of the scorpion is poisonous, snakes bite hard. I am afraid of the dark. It is like I can't see, and I am afraid I am going to bump into something scary."

Roberto was allergic to most formulas from birth. He had to go on a predigested formula. On the other formulas he would get very hungry, and when he went to suck, he would start to cramp and cry.

"We always fight over getting him to eat. Every mealtime, especially in the morning. He does like chocolate cake and will eat that in the morning. But not much else."

Roberto has always vomited with certain smells he finds offensive, like cat poop. He gets frequent coughs with colds and can be up all night coughing and gagging.

Roberto goes to Catholic school and recently got a Bible picture book. He was immediately fascinated by the picture of the devil. His cousin recently said something about hell and Roberto repeated it. He started asking questions like, "What is hell? Who lives there? Why do you go there?" At Halloween he asked about skulls. He ended up being Dracula last Halloween and wanted to know why they came out at night and why they are cold. He said, "I am not going there (to hell), bad people go there. "I asked again about his dreams and he said, "The scariest thing is the devil is cutting off my head."

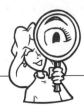

Curious Clues

Looking for a clue to Roberto's symptoms, I searched the repertory for the symptom "aversion to food, in general, in the morning." Only six remedies—not much to go on. Then I noticed one of the remedies was Mancinella, which has ideations about the devil, fears and dreams of the devil, of being taken by the devil, and fears of evil and the dark.

Roberto's case was difficult because there was no clear reason why he was such a picky eater, so sensitive to foods and smells, and gagged so easily. The worst time for Roberto was in the morning when he seemed to have no appetite.

I gave Roberto the plant remedy Mancinella (or Manganeel Apple) in the *Euphorbiacae* family. Patients needing this remedy have a strong sensitivity to odors and a tendency to gag with nausea as well as violent headaches. The remedy picture also includes a strong desire for salt, and Roberto, when he was allowed to eat junk food, would always go for chips. He never gagged from chips!

On follow-up one month later, Roberto's mother reported he wasn't having any more headaches. There had been no vomiting and very little gagging. While he still won't sit at the table with the others, he has tried many new things and likes some of them. His teacher was impressed that he was eating a snack and lunch at school, which he would seldom do before the remedy. He has also stopped complaining of stomachaches. He still likes tomatoes but the craving (which was quite large, often eating four or five per day) had decreased. His mother said, "He has let go of the devil." She hadn't heard him speak of that fear in several weeks.

Roberto's mother wrote me eight months later to let me know that "Roberto has been in good health all winter with no coughs. He is now eating better and trying new things all the time."

Bed-Wetting

Nocturnal enuresis, commonly called bed-wetting, affects approximately 30 percent of children at age four, 10 percent at six years old, 3 percent at age 12, and 1 percent at age 18 years. At various ages, children learn to use the toilet during the day and later are able to sleep through the night without loss of bladder control. Bed-wetting is more common in boys than girls, tends to run in families, crowded households, and in homes where there's a smoker.

Bed-wetting is usually cured by time, and the development of bladder control at night comes naturally with maturity. Most of the time, it is not a willful act, and punishment is never a good solution. Up to age six, there is a high spontaneous cure rate, while each year after six years old, the cure falls 15 percent per year. Treatment is usually not warranted until after age six, when embarrassment becomes a prime motivator. Counseling your child about some healthy bedtime habits is a common approach. Get them involved so that they feel empowered during a time when they may experience shame, blame, or guilt. Have them join in by avoiding drinking fluids two to three hours before going to bed, record wet and dry nights, and change clothing and bedding when wet. Positive reinforcement for dry nights and reassurance that all will be well soon are important facts to remember during these often trying and frustrating times.

Homeopathic treatment can be a safe and effective treatment to speed up the natural process or treat an underlying condition, whether physical or emotional, that contributes to your child's bed-wetting.

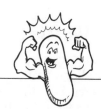

Potent Pellets

Most children are trained for bowel control between the ages of two and three and for urinary control between the ages of three and four. By age five years, the average child can go to the toilet alone. About 30 percent of normal four-year olds and 10 percent of six-year olds have not achieved nighttime bladder control.

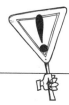

Caution Keeper

Be concerned about bed-wetting, but only if your child is older than six and has never been dry at night, continues to wet the bed at least twice a month, or suddenly begins wetting at night or during the day after a period of having been dry. Consult your primary care provider to rule out conditions such as bladder and kidney infections or diabetes.

The next story will illustrate how homeopathy made a real contribution to the health and happiness of a bed-wetting child.

Bed-Wetting Case (Presented by Pamela J. Herring)

Briana was a popular and vivacious girl with lots of friends. She had been coming in for homeopathic treatment since she was two years old, and had responded very well to remedies for her temper tantrums and nightmares. When she had not stopped wetting the bed by age three to four, her mother began to be concerned. By five years old, Briana was beginning to have sleepovers with her friends and was becoming self-conscious about the problem. She was timid at times and still had a bit of a temper, becoming angry very quickly. Her mother said she would fly off the handle after getting worked up and would even make things up to be angry at, saying she is the "mad pony." Then she would lash out physically, even at adults. Briana would get jealous if she felt one of her friends was prettier or had more than she had materially. Briana was given the homeopathic remedy Sepia.

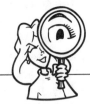

Curious Clues

The unique properties of Briana's story were considered and I chose to give her the homeopathic remedy Sepia. I've listed the characteristics that helped me decide on this remedy in the form that you would use when looking them up in a homeopathic repertory, which is listed by categories (see Chapter 8, "Your First Visit to a Homeopath"):

➤ Mind; anger, irascibility; tendency

➤ Mind; anger, irascibility; tendency; violent

➤ Mind; delusions, imaginations

➤ Mind; irritability

➤ Mind; jealousy; children; between

➤ Mind; timidity

➤ Bladder; urination; involuntary; children, in

As has often happened in treating bed-wetting, the nightly problem stopped within 24 hours. Over the next two years, she was given several doses of Sepia whenever she had the occasional relapses of either the bed-wetting or irritability.

ADD and ADD with Hyperactivity: The Attention Dimension

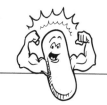

Confusion, controversy, and constant challenges abound when a family suspects its child may have attention deficit disorder, or ADD. *The Diagnostic and Statistical Manual of Mental Disorders (DSM-IV)* defines attention deficit disorder as a persistent and frequent pattern of developmentally inappropriate attention and impulsivity, with or without hyperactivity. Most parents tell me they saw signs of this when their child was an infant. They may have seen overexcitability, brief or no attention spans when playing with toys, and noticeable differences in motor development than their child's peers. ADD or ADD with hyperactivity is usually not formally diagnosed before age four because these signs could be part of normal development, and they could "grow out of it."

Confusion and conflict occur when examining the statistics during the evolution of our understanding this condition. Statistics say that 5 percent to 20 percent of school-age children have ADD, and from 10 percent to 60 percent of childhood onset ADD will continue into adulthood. These are big gaps in statistics. The condition is thought to occur more frequently in families—suggesting its genetic connection, but no clear reason why ADD or ADD with hyperactivity exists has been determined. ADD with hyperactivity is diagnosed 10 times more frequently in boys, but there is growing concern that girls may be getting overlooked, because their lack of attention (ADD) does not "disrupt the classroom." The children may have normal or even high intelligence.

> **Potent Pellets**
>
> An estimated 5 percent to 10 percent of school-aged children are affected with attention deficit disorder, or ADD, accounting for half of the childhood referrals to diagnostic clinics. ADD with hyperactivity is seen 10 times more frequently in boys than in girls.
>
> *Source:* The Merck Manual, 17th Edition

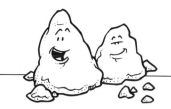

> **Natural Nuggets**
>
> Make sure your school tests your child for learning disabilities if you observe him getting stuck in schoolwork. At least 30 percent of children with ADD may also suffer from learning disabilities. Conditions such as dyslexia do not respond to medication and may need additional educational assistance.

Diagnosing ADD/ADHD

Diagnosing ADD/ADHD is primarily done through observable signs. Less than 5 percent of children with ADD/ADD with hyperactivity have symptoms and signs of neurological disorders. Hypotheses of why these symptoms occur include neurotransmitter

131

abnormalities in dopaminergic and moradrenergic systems, toxins, neurologic immaturity, infections, drug exposure during pregnancy, head injuries, and other environmental factors.

DSM-IV Criteria for ADD

Signs of inattention

Often fails to pay close attention to details

Difficulty sustaining attention at work or play

Does not seem to listen when spoken to directly

Often does not follow through on instructions and fails to finish tasks

Has difficulty organizing tasks and activities

Often avoids, dislikes, or is reluctant to engage in tasks that require sustained mental efforts

Often loses things

Easily distracted by outside stimuli

Often forgetful

Hyperactivity

Often fidgets with hands or feet, or squirms

Frequently leaves seat in classroom and elsewhere

Runs about or climbs excessively

Has difficulty playing quietly

Is often on the go or acts as if "driven by a motor"

Talks excessively

Impulsivity

Blurts out answers before questions have been completed

Difficulty waiting their turn

Often interrupts or intrudes on others

Follow-up studies show that children with ADD/ADHD do not outgrow their difficulties. Problems in adolescence and adulthood show in areas such as academic failure, low self-esteem, and difficulty learning appropriate social behavior. Without proper treatment, the symptoms still exist, but may be better hidden as an adult through antisocial behavior. I often hear adults say, "That's just how I am" as they limit their real potential by walling off the areas and people that challenge their behavioral issues.

Treatment of ADD/ADHD: The Ritalin Rocket

Conventional medicine currently recommends psychostimulant drugs combined with counseling for best results in controlling symptoms. There is a growing concern that many children are being poorly diagnosed and given drugs without education or counseling services, which show some improvement for only less-impulsive ADD children who have stable home environments. Children with poor impulse control are helped less by drug treatment.

Here are some side effects of methylphenidate (generic Ritalin):

➤ Sleep disturbance

➤ Headache

➤ Appetite suppression

➤ Elevated blood pressure

➤ Depression

➤ Stomachache

➤ Growth reduction

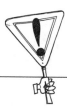

Caution Keeper

Many conditions other than ADD/ADD with hyperactivity can have learning problems. Make sure you have your child's learning and vision checked. The stress of moving, death in the family, parental job loss, or divorce can trigger changes in behavior such as depression, anxiety, or other serious emotional problems that may mimic ADD/ADD with hyperactivity. Consult with your care provider for a thorough evaluation.

There are growing controversies about teaching our children to pop pills to solve their problems, while de-emphasizing their role in participating in awareness, family structure, and behavior modification. This concern has been fueled by the recent abuse that Ritalin has experienced. High school and college students are using Ritalin to party with their friends. The Drug Enforcement Administration (DEA) identifies Ritalin as one of the top-10 controlled drugs that are frequently reported stolen. It's sold on the street as "Vitamin R" and "R-Ball." In many cities, Ritalin abuse moved from the club scene and is now available to younger adolescents in social situations billed as "no alcohol" events according to Paul Ulrich, a Chicago-based DEA spokesman. There are also reports of parents popping the drug from their own kid's supplies, hoping it will help with weight loss or give them an energy boost. Ritalin is a slow-acting drug, so pills are crushed and snorted or injected for a quicker high.

Homeopathic care can be an effective treatment that may reduce or eliminate the need for drug treatment. I recommend that parents use homeopathic care along with the recommended counseling, consistent parenting techniques, home structure, and well-defined limits. Homeopathics help your child to break free of a cycle of behavior that challenges your whole family.

ADD with Hyperactivity: Sweet or Sour! (Presented by Savitri Clarke)

Tony walks into my office looking very wary, clearly unsure of what is to come. He is scratching his arms, which are covered with a dry, red, painful-looking rash. When I ask him about school, he says, "I am supposed to go into the fourth grade but my mother made me stay back." He is unhappy about this. He feels it has nothing to do with him.

As I try to talk with Tony, he is bouncing up and down in his chair. His mother tells me, "He has had eczema all over his body since birth. He also had ear infections and got tubes." He, his two sisters, and his mother all have food allergies. As Tony continues to scratch, I ask him if he scratches much at night. "No, only once," he says. This seems unbelievable and I notice his mother rolling her eyes. Tony tells me he gets mad at his sister when she scratches him with her toes but denies ever hitting her.

At this point, Tony's mother asks his father to leave the room with Tony so she can talk with me privately. She tells me of her anxiety and stress during the pregnancy, when, as a senior in high school, she had to live with her brother because her parents had moved away. "Now Tony's father puts him down and belittles him in front of other people. He does the same thing to me and the other kids. He spanks them hard. Tony hears what his father says to me and repeats it, treating me poorly. I am trying to hold the family together but don't know how much longer I can do it. There is nothing any of us can do to please his father."

Tony's mother tells me Tony is very impulsive and swears a lot.

At this point, Tony and his father join us again. Tony is not happy to be here, is extremely anxious and restless, and keeps looking at his father as if he is waiting for something bad to happen. Tony has been in two residential programs, neither of which seemed to help him. He is very unfocused at school. He is on a medication to help him focus but it doesn't help much. He still speaks out of turn and is easily distracted. He won't do anything unless you bribe him. His self-esteem is very low. There have been many occasions where he has taken pencils and pens from other kids or has taken money from his parents' room. When he gets mad, he often stamps his feet.

One of the most disturbing things about Tony is that he often hits his sisters for no apparent reason. He gets picked on at school and tends to run away. He feels people are picking on him all the time. His mother adds, "He has no conscience and he shows no remorse for anything he does. What scares me is he doesn't seem to feel anything even when he hurts someone."

Every time I asked Tony a question, he would look at me as if clearly assessing what I wanted him to say and then he would try to say it. He was clearly lying, as if by lying he could avoid getting into trouble, getting hurt. He could be sweet or perform a hurtful act without any feelings of regret.

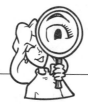

Curious Clues

Tony was given Anacardium, the Marking Nut. This is a remedy for people who have very low self-esteem, often from continued abuse. It has proved very useful in many cases of schizophrenia. The symptoms indicating Anacardium were ...

➤ Suspicious

➤ Impulsive

➤ Restlessness with anxiety

➤ Disobedient

➤ Delusion (feeling) injured

➤ Swears

➤ Want of moral feeling

➤ Stamps his feet

➤ Steals

➤ Lies

➤ Violent

➤ Difficulty studying due to anxiety

➤ Delusion (the split of the personality)

After two months, Tony's mother brought him back. He was noticeably calmer and actually looked me in the eye, which he wouldn't do before. When I asked him if he had been scratching at night (the same question I asked him last time), he said, "At night is the worst time but overall it is much better!" I was thrilled to get my first honest answer out of Tony and felt he was on the road to recovery. His mother offered, "Tony is slowly getting better at school. He seems to be developing a conscience so he is not striking out as much and often feels bad when he does. He is getting into trouble less now because he is less impulsive and can think things through."

Over the next year Tony continued to improve. His eczema was almost gone and caused little discomfort. I was impressed by how much he had improved emotionally. Whether you are a family member or health-care provider, ADD/ADD with hyperactivity requires patience and persistence for successful outcomes. I believe we owe our children the best choices of treatment that will set the course for their entire lives. Cooperation, communication, and follow-through are key elements in whatever methods you decide to use. I hope you will consult with a qualified homeopathic in your area to explore this valuable treatment option.

Next I'll take you on a tour of the maze of motherly concerns that confront women including fertility issues, morning sickness, labor pains, and postpartum depression.

The Least You Need to Know

➤ Many of the most debilitating childhood emotional conditions can be effectively treated with homeopathic remedies.

➤ Fear of embarrassment and stigmas still motivate individuals to conceal their emotional challenges.

➤ Homeopathic medicines offer treatment by restoring complete health with swift and mild methods using sound time-tested principles.

➤ Parental challenges of anxiety-induced stomachache, obsessive-compulsive disorder, and fussy eating can be successfully treated with safe, nonhabit-forming homeopathic remedies.

➤ ADD and ADHD symptoms do not improve with age. Homeopathic treatment combined with other behavior modifications and counseling can offer sound relief for both children and adults.

Part 3

Putting Out Fires

I refer to emergency care as "forest fire medicine." When a patient calls me, I parachute into the blaze that is encompassing his or her life. As a team, we pull together our resources, do our best to contain the blaze, minimize damage, and begin to plant the seeds for recovery and wellness.

We'll look at the healing potential that homeopathy offers to household emergencies such as burns, stings, and bites, as well as flu symptoms, food poisoning, fractures, and wounds. We'll examine the fiery frustrations of menopause and painful periods, infertility, morning sickness, labor pains, and postpartum depression. The air can get smoky, so hold onto your homeopathic knowledge when treating asthma, coughs, sore throats, and sinuses.

We'll consider skin problems such as acne, eczema, psoriasis, and poison ivy to discover how homeopathic medicine helps stimulate the healing of the often painful and embarrassing terrain of our bodies.

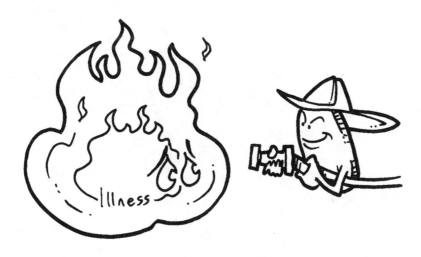

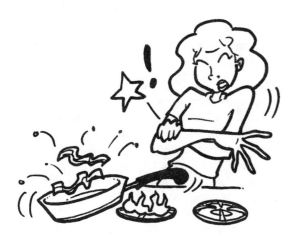

Chapter 13

Emergency Homeopathic Care

Anyone who has ever dealt with accidental injuries knows they demand our immediate attention. Conditions accompanied by pain, vomiting, or itchy rashes also require fast action and speedy recovery. Homeopathic remedies are probably best known in this country for their safe treatment of acute or traumatic injuries. In this chapter, you'll learn the differences and similarities between acute and chronic care with homeopathic medicines. We'll also learn how these diluted medicines can effectively treat such common traumatic concerns as burns, stings, fractures, and acute wounds.

Flus and food poisoning with their exhausting symptoms of fever, nausea, vomiting, and diarrhea can be significantly relieved by boosting your body's immunity and natural healing ability through the use of homeopathic medicines.

Homeopathic Treatment of Acute vs. Chronic Conditions

In general, we think of *acute* situations—whether they are medical or not—as being immediate, possibly severe, but usually of short duration. The word *chronic* conjures up thoughts of long-lasting occurrences; something that keeps coming back with more time being involved. This is the case with illness as well. We expect more severity, but less time to experience it with acute injuries, while chronic conditions keep coming back to us like boomerangs, usually with less severe symptoms but with a pesky persistence.

Although acute and chronic conditions have different qualities and time duration of symptoms, the best homeopathic care still involves treating all aspects of the individual. Remember the last family crisis? Think of the individuals in your family and how each one dealt with the stress of the situation. The person who the crisis actually happened to may not react with the intensity of a frightened family onlooker. What about those who get mad, feel rejected, sad, worry all the time that it might happen again? The totality of symptoms that include the physical, mental, and emotional experiences of the individual still form the most complete picture to match with a homeopathic remedy.

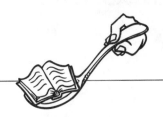

Dose of Info

Samuel Hahnemann defines acute and chronic illness in paragraph 72 of *The Organon* (O'Reilly, 1996): **Acute** diseases are rapid illnesses; processes of the abnormally mistuned life principle which are suited to complete their course more or less quickly; **chronic** diseases are those which (each in its own way) dynamically mistune the living organism with small, often unnoticed beginnings.

Many over-the-counter homeopathic products list only a couple of symptoms, which are often superficial qualities of a remedy. Patients will often tell me, "I've tried homeopathy before, and it didn't work." Cutting back on the accuracy of prescribing by being unfamiliar with the whole picture increases the odds of missing the mark and being less than satisfied with your therapeutic results. Sometimes you get lucky and choose a remedy that works very well, but when you go back to use it again, it doesn't work. Did the remedy change? Recognizing the total symptoms of an individual, whether for an acute or chronic condition, is still the most effective way to ensure accuracy and satisfaction with your homeopathic remedy choices.

Arnica: Choosin' for a Bruisin'

Arnica Montana grows up to two feet in the mountainous regions of Europe and western North America. The orange-yellow flower has been referred to as mountain tobacco, Leopard's Bane or Wolf's Bane, but is commonly called Arnica. An estimated 300 Arnica-containing tinctures, ointments, and homeopathic remedies are manufactured for the German market alone!

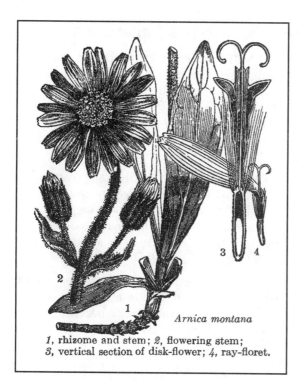

Arnica montana

1, rhizome and stem; *2*, flowering stem;
3, vertical section of disk-flower; *4*, ray-floret.

Arnica is one of the most well-known homeopathic products commonly used for soothing sore muscles and reducing pain and inflammation. This physical complaint is usually accompanied by patients experiencing a fixed idea that they are quite well, despite a serious injury.

Arnica should not be used topically on broken skin or wounds, but has been approved by the Commission E, the German Regulatory Authority similar to our own FDA, for indications including ...

➤ Fever and colds.

➤ Inflammation of the skin.

➤ Cough/bronchitis.

➤ Inflammation of the mouth and larynx.

➤ Rheumatism.

➤ Common cold.

➤ Blunt injuries.

➤ Tendency to infection.

Source: PDR for Herbal Medicines, 2nd Edition

Homeopathic Arnica is often used with any type of trauma, while its best uses arise out of the total symptoms of the patient, which may include cardiac pain, fear of heart disease, irritability, and a desire to be alone. In case of serious injuries, patients who may benefit from Arnica often believe they are well and do not need a doctor or anyone's help. Using the full range of symptoms assures the greatest accuracy and effectiveness when choosing Arnica.

141

Stings and Bites: The Puncture Juncture

Do you get a little jumpy when you hear the unmistakable buzzing of bees, hornets, wasps, or yellow jackets? Being stung is painful, but for those who are allergic to insects, the severe reaction is terrifying. According to the National Institute of Allergy and Infectious Disease (NIAID), more than 500,000 people visit emergency rooms every year for allergic reactions to insect stings. The same organization states that at least 40 Americans die each year from severe allergic reactions to insect bites.

You can apply ice to most bites and stings to reduce the localized swelling and time will fix the rest. If you have an allergic reaction, you should immediately consult emergency medical care. Many people who know they have severe allergies to stings and bites carry an auto injector of epinephrine (adrenaline), which can be a life-saving tool. Using an auto injector should be followed by an immediate trip to urgent care.

Homeopathic medicines are a safe treatment for the pain, swelling, and mild-to-moderate allergic reaction. They are not a substitute for emergency care during severe allergic reactions.

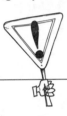

Caution Keeper

Once you've been stung and experience an allergic reaction, you have a 60 percent chance of developing a similar or worse reaction if stung again.

Source: American College of Allergy, Asthma, and Immunology

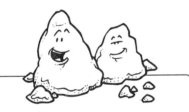

Natural Nuggets

If you are stung by an insect, remove the stinger by scraping or flicking at it with your fingernail or a credit card. Do not pull or squeeze the stinger because you could release more venom into your skin.

Jellyfish Stings—A Fishy Story

My wife and I were on our first anniversary cruising in the Caribbean. We love the clear blue view when you dive or snorkel in these waters and had decided to snorkel with a group off the island of Martinique.

The captain said we could find a spectacular view by swimming through a tight channel and popping out into a hidden lagoon that opened up to the sky. Three of us left the pack to swim into an opening in the rock forged by years of pounding surf. All we thought we had to do was catch a ride from the tide. With mask and fins in place, I launched toward the opening, only to be met at the entrance by a large school of silver-dollar-sized jellyfish. I smashed into them so fast I barely had time to cover my face with my hands as numerous little stings and zings covered my upper body. Once inside, we had all been stung, we were frightened, and we didn't exactly fully appreciate this pricey view. The problem was we had to go out the same way we came in. We boosted each other with courage and swam through the jellyfish feeding line to the boat.

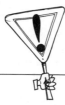

Caution Keeper

Typical signs of an allergic reaction to a bite or sting include hives (red swollen areas on your skin that may be itchy), swelling or itching on sites other than where you were stung, difficulty breathing, a swollen tongue, and a hoarse voice. Bites from most spiders and insects are of little danger. The irritation is from the injection of salivary fluid or venom into the skin that provokes a small itchy swelling typically lasting a few hours or days.

My face, arms, and chest were covered with growing red, raised, and itchy burning hives. When I arrived onshore, I found that the heat of the sun aggravated the itching, and I felt better in the air-conditioning of our room or when I applied ice. I was beginning to worry as I experienced some mild difficulty in breathing and a growing fear that something was terribly wrong; what if I died? I opened up a small homeopathic travel kit that I take with me and took Apis, the highly diluted venom of a bumblebee.

I took a dose of Apis every half hour for about three hours. My skin started to cool and the burning subsided. By the time dinner was served, the redness, itching, and swelling were noticeably improved. Although tired, I regained my honeymoon spirit. I checked on my fellow adventurers who had already been to see the ship's doctor and were in their cabins. My wife and I headed for the conga line!

Curious Clues

I used Apis 6c on my Caribbean crisis, mainly because that's the only potency I had. At the time, I felt the totality of my symptoms reflected Apis by these symptoms:

➤ Rash with burning pains
➤ Swelling, better from cold or cold applications
➤ Red, itching skin
➤ Active, busy people
➤ Irritability
➤ Fear of death
➤ Stinging pains with swelling

Food Poisoning: Forget the Seconds, Please

It's a summertime car trip, wheeling your way cross-country, seeing the sights and driving where the wind takes you. Stopping off midafternoon for a bite to eat sounds good, maybe something light from the salad bar. Moments like this should ring all the warning bells: You could be trading in a Grand Canyon vista for the sights and sounds of a motel bathroom. Salmonella, caued by

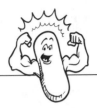

Potent Pellets

More than two million Americans report illnesses that are traced to foods they have eaten. Food poisoning and stomach flus are both inflammations of the stomach and intestines but the similarities end there. Food poisoning is usually caused by bacteria that have multiplied in food or drink; the bacteria produce toxins that make you sick. Stomach flus are caused by viruses passed directly from person to person.

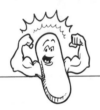

Potent Pellets

In India, when there is an epidemic of diarrhea and/or vomiting and there is neither time nor resources to take complete cases, the homeopaths give Arsenicum Album as the first prescription. It is reported to be effective in over 50 percent of such cases! If that doesn't work, they take a more complete case.

Staphylococcus aureus, accounts for about 25 percent of all cases of food poisoning and is commonly found in the nose and throat. Food products—such as a salad bar without protective coverings—can become contaminated if they are coughed or sneezed on.

Salmonella is most often found in meat, poultry, egg products, tuna, macaroni, and potato salads. If the salad bar at your next noontime meal does not look fresh, you could be headed toward a salmonella salad that is typically followed by diarrhea, nausea, vomiting, abdominal cramps, and fatigue, usually two to eight hours after eating contaminated food.

Here are the symptoms of food poisoning:

➤ **Bacterial food poisoning**: Abdominal cramps, diarrhea, and vomiting starting one hour to four days after tainted food, lasting up to four days.

➤ **Viral food poisoning**: Vomiting, diarrhea, abdominal cramps, headaches, fever, and chills; beginning 12 to 48 hours after eating contaminated foods, especially seafood.

➤ **Chemical food poisoning**: Vomiting, diarrhea, sweating, dizziness, tearing of eyes, excessive salivation, mental confusion, and stomach pain beginning about 30 minutes after eating bad food.

➤ **Botulism**: Partial loss of speech or vision, muscle paralysis from the head down, and vomiting may indicate this rare type of food poisoning.

Food poisoning is extremely uncomfortable and will ruin a weekend getaway or an island honeymoon for sure! Rest and keeping fluids down are the standard conventional prescription. If you have a medical condition such as AIDS, diabetes, or cancer that may challenge your immune system, then the effects of food poisoning may be more serious.

If you notice ground-coffee-colored blood in your vomit or diarrhea, dehydration (crying without tears, dry mouth, no saliva, no sweat with a fever), uncontrollable vomiting or diarrhea, dizziness, or confusion that do not go away after a couple of days, you should call your health-care provider.

Homeopathic treatments of food poisoning may offer significant relief and shorten the time with symptoms during the difficult and painful disorder.

Food Poisoning (Presented by Savitri Clarke)

It was a warm quiet Sunday morning when I got an emergency call from my patient John, who was away on vacation and very sick. He pleaded, "Please, you must help me. I feel like I'm going to die or maybe I want to! It must have been the meat in the lasagna last night. I woke up at 1 A.M. with horrible cramping and nausea. It wasn't long before the vomiting started. By the time the vomiting turned to dry heaves, the diarrhea started. I can't believe there was that much fluid in me!"

John sounded very anxious. I could hear from his voice that he was pacing while he was talking. I asked him some questions about how he felt and what made him feel better or worse. He responded, "I am very restless and need to move even though I think that makes the cramping and diarrhea worse. When the diarrhea kicks in, it feels like a hot poker moving through my intestines. There is some relief after a bout of diarrhea, but then the cycle starts again. I am freezing and can't seem to get warm. I am getting really weak and now I sweat when I walk from one side of the room to the other. I have my homeopathic emergency kit with me. Please tell me what to take *now!*"

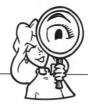

Curious Clues

John appeared to have a classic case of food poisoning. While most of the symptoms of his vomiting and diarrhea where not very striking, there were some distinguishing characteristics of John's condition:

- ➤ Anxiety, fear of death
- ➤ Sensation of hot poker moving through intestines
- ➤ Weakness
- ➤ Chilliness
- ➤ Restlessness
- ➤ Perspiration with slight exertion
- ➤ Pleading, begging

The remedy chosen on the basis of these distinguishing symptoms was Arsenicum Album, or white arsenic.

I told John to start taking the Arsenicum from his kit and to repeat a dose every one to four hours as needed. He phoned 24 hours later to say he was better almost immediately after beginning the remedy, his anxiety lessened, and within 30 minutes he was able to rest without any recurrence of the vomiting or diarrhea. John could continue to enjoy his vacation.

Fractures: My Achy, Breaky Bones

Fractures most often occur from a number of occurrences such as traumas from sport's injuries, car accidents, or slips and falls. A growing number of fractures are caused from osteoporosis, where bones become less dense and more brittle. This is an increasing concern for men and women over the age of 60. In a June 22, 2000, interview, Douglas Bauer, professor of medicine, epidemiology, and biostatistics at the University of California in San Francisco, stated that osteoporosis affects one in three women and one in ten men. Professor Bauer went on to say that 20 percent of individuals with hip fractures (an estimated 200,000 people) die within a year, and that many more never return to independent living. He estimates that about half of women over 50 years of age will have a fracture due to osteoporosis sometime during their life.

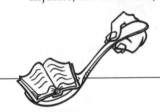

Dose of Info

A **fracture** is a break or crack in a bone. If the skin over the bone remains intact, it is referred to as a closed or simple fracture. If the bone breaks through the skin, it is named an open or compound fracture.

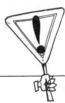

Caution Keeper

A new study finds that teenage girls who drink lots of soda may be more prone to bone fractures and osteoporosis than girls who do not. Between 40 percent and 60 percent of peak bone mass is built during teenage years. The large amounts of phosphorus in colas interfere with the absorption of calcium. According to the study, teens have doubled or tripled their consumption of soft drinks while cutting back on milk by 40 percent. Girls who drank soft drinks were three times more likely to sustain a bone fracture.

Source: Children's Hospital of Long Island Jewish Medical Center

Osteoporosis and fractures related to this condition cost about $13.8 billion a year and affect between 25 million and 30 million American adults. Conventional care calls for prompt medical attention for diagnostics and casting. Homeopathy complements the process of healing and as you will see can help boost your body's ability to heal a stubborn fracture.

Nonhealing Fracture (Presented by Savitri Clarke)

Sam came to see me quite concerned about the status of his right lower leg. He had been in an automobile accident seven months before and had suffered a compound fracture of the right tibia and fibula. The leg had been in a cast all this time and according to x-rays, the bones did not appear to be knitting properly. There was some concern that another surgery might be necessary to rebreak the bones and reset them.

After talking with Sam for a while it was clear that he was a healthy 45-year-old man. His only symptom was the failure of his broken leg to heal properly. This seemed a clear case for the remedy Symphytum, or homeopathic comfrey ("bone-set"). It was necessary to take a complete case first because there are many other remedies that could have been a better fit. I recommended that Sam take a low potency of Symphytum daily for a month.

Sam took the remedy and was pleased to see the bones completely healed on the x-ray at the end of one month. His physician removed the cast and Sam was able to start the process of strengthening his right leg. Once again, the right remedy stimulated the body to heal itself!

Influenza: The Scare in the Air

Influenza, or "flu" as it is commonly referred to, is an extremely contagious viral disease that appears most frequently in the winter and early spring.

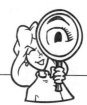

Curious Clues

The root of the comfrey plant contains a crystalline solid that stimulates the growth of bone cells, a useful remedy for injuries to bones, cartilages, and periosteum (a thin sheath covering bone) with excessive pain. It can also be helpful with painful old injuries as well as stitching pain that remains after a wound is healed. Symphytum is also useful for injuries to the eyeball, especially when caused by a blunt instrument.

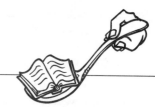

Dose of Info

Influenza literally means *influence* in Italian; this term was used in the 1500s when people thought the quick spread of illness was caused by the "influence" of the stars and plants. The name was commonly used following a severe epidemic that struck Italy in 1743 and spread throughout Europe.

Flu symptoms affect the upper respiratory tract and are easily spread to other people by coughing- and sneezing-infected airborne water droplets, which spray onto us and contaminate objects we touch, like desks, chairs, and countertops. The initial symptoms of the flu can be mistaken for a common cold, with the familiar headache, fatigue, and body aches. In most cases of flu, fever develops, which distinguishes it from a cold. You may experience high fever, alternating with uncontrollable chills, sore throat, dry hacking cough, nasal congestion, sneezing, and headaches. Most of us have had the flu (a group of influenza viruses A, B, and C), and will know that you get weak and don't feel like doing or eating anything.

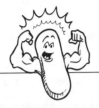

Potent Pellets

Today influenza and its complications are fatal to about 200,000 Americans each year. The global influenza epidemic of 1918, which started in a military training camp in Kansas, killed more than 500,000 people in the United States.

Influenza is rarely dangerous to healthy individuals. The spread of the virus usually begins with school-age children who bring home the virus and infect their families, who then share it with friends and fellow workers. Because the virus does weaken your immune system, it can make you more susceptible to pneumonia, ear infections, and sinus trouble. Among people over 65 years of age, serious respiratory infections like pneumonia could result.

The usual treatment for the aches and pains of the flu is to take aspirin, drink plenty of water, and bed rest until your fever subsides for a couple of days. Prevention has been commonly done with vaccinations, but with an estimated 200 different cold and flu viruses, which are constantly changing yearly, prevention has been only partially successful. That's why flu shots are only good for one year.

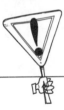

Caution Keeper

Most flu vaccines are made in egg products. If you have and allergic reaction to eggs, the vaccine may cause serious allergic reactions. Check with your health-care provider for other side effects of the flu vaccinations that are recommended for you.

Homeopathic care helps your body heal during a flu when your immune system is struggling to fight off the virus and restore health. In the next patient's story, you will see why these tiny pellets can be a powerful ally in feeling better and regaining your health during the flu season.

Flu (Presented by Savitri Clarke)

Jason phoned and seemed upset when he was told he would have to wait an hour, as I was with a patient. When I later phoned Jason, he told me the following story:

"Yesterday morning I woke up with a slight fever and aching all over. I thought it was just a little virus so I went to work. By noon my fever had risen to 101° and the body aches were much worse so I came home. I couldn't even read because just the movement of my eyeballs caused such pain. I got into bed and stayed as still as I could. Anytime I moved everything hurt more. It even hurts when I laugh! My head started to pound and it felt like it would burst."

This was the second day of what seemed like a painful case of the flu. I asked Jason for any other information about his condition or anything that affects how he feels. "I am so dry. My lips are peeling and I can't seem to quench my thirst. I am drinking ice water by the glass full but I can't seem to get enough. I keep snapping at my wife who I know is just trying to help. Everything she does annoys me. I just want to be left alone."

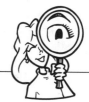

Curious Clues

The clues clearly pointed toward the remedy Bryonia. The important Bryonia characteristics seemed to be ...

➤ Pain aggravated by any movement, even the eyes.

➤ Bursting head pain.

➤ Dryness, lips peeling.

➤ Great thirst for large quantities frequently.

➤ Irritability.

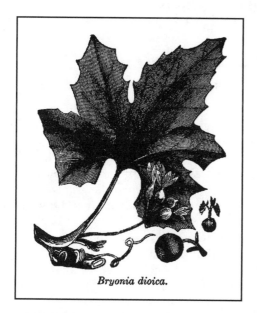

Bryonia dioica.

Bryonia is indicated for flu relief with symptoms that include pain made worse from any movement, bursting headache, dryness, peeling lips, irritability with great thirst, drinking large amounts of water frequently.

When I looked at how Jason was manifesting his flu symptoms, I recommended that Jason take the remedy Bryonia, or homeopathic wild hops. All of his symptoms were keynotes of this remedy. Just to confirm the remedy choice, I asked him if he found the parts of his body that he was lying on to be more or less painful than the other parts. He said, surprisingly, that the parts that were against the bed felt better. This is another keynote of Bryonia, feeling better from pressure or lying on the painful side. So I recommended that Jason take a dose of Bryonia every two to six hours depending on the intensity of his symptoms and to call me after 24 hours. When he phoned the next day he said, "That was amazing. Within an hour of taking the first dose the aching subsided and my mood improved. It was a good thing because my wife had just about had it with me!" He just felt a little tired but felt he could return to work the next day. Jason had a previous pattern of having flus go into his chest with a long recovery. He was thrilled to have nipped this one in the bud!

Burns: The Degrees of Discomfort

Your skin is the largest sensitive living tissue of your body, composed of three primary layers: the epidermis, dermis, and subcutaneous. Exposure to heat above 120°F will damage these cells and cause some degree of burning. We automatically think of fire with burns; remember that electrical and chemical burns are included in the causes of the more than two million people who get burns in the United States every year. Of those, 300,000 are burned seriously, 70,000 require admission to a hospital, and 6,000 die from their injuries. Children and the elderly are more susceptible to more serious forms of burns because their skin is thinner.

The remedy Cantharis is homeopathic Spanish fly. It is useful in first-degree burns with (or before) blisters with burning pain relieved by cold applications of this product.

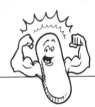

Potent Pellets

In the 1899 edition of *Merck's Manual* for physicians, there are numerous solutions for wound care outlined including the use of blotting paper (used to soak up extra ink when writing with a fountain pen) soaked in analgesics such as Bismuth Subgallate. It is recommended that this be applied externally on wounds, ulcers, and eczemas.

Acute First-Degree Burns (Presented by Savitri Clarke)

We were visiting friends for a barbecue with our four-year old son, Kailin. He was happily playing with our friends' children as we stood around in the yard talking to our hosts. The kettle grill was heating up and soon we would smell that lovely aroma of fresh fish and vegetables. Just when the grill was hot and ready to go, Kailin got too close to it and touched the bottom of the kettle with his elbow. I saw it happen in a flash but was too far away to stop it. I ran to him as he screamed in pain and saw a large patch of skin already changing color. Luckily, I knew these friends had just that week purchased a homeopathic home kit. I told them to get it quickly as I held my ice-filled glass on his arm, which helped the pain a little. Within a couple of minutes the kit arrived and I chose the remedy Cantharis and gave Kailin a dose. Within two or three minutes the pain stopped and we all watched over the next 15 minutes as the skin started to lighten in color.

I repeated the remedy several times, whenever he said the pain was starting to return. By the next day the burn was all but gone and totally cleared in two days. We were all amazed that no blisters ever formed. Never were we more happy to have friends who also believed in homeopathy!

Wound Care: A Cutting Remark

Even a paper cut will send me yelping around looking for sympathy, let alone the more serious slashes, punctures, and wounds that can occur. Severity is usually the key that sends us flying to the emergency room or breaking open our own first-aid kit and attempting a home treatment.

People who have diabetes and blood vessel disease such as partially blocked arteries and veins may have extra concern over nonhealing wounds. Chronic skin infections, vascular diseases, skin cancer, immobilization, and poor nutrition are also linked to stubborn or nonhealing wounds. Proper diet and nutrition can significantly contribute to the healing of a traumatic injury, postoperative recovery, or chronic nonhealing wounds.

Most hospitals have special wound-care centers where techniques such as special dressings, low-strength electrical-field stimulators, cultured skin substitute, and DNA growth therapy are practiced.

Homeopathic medicines can be a wonderful addition to a comprehensive wound management team. The next scenario will show you an all-out emergency that was greatly alleviated by the use of homeopathy.

Acute Injury (Presented by Pamela J. Herring)

My good friend Carol called me when she got back from a ski trip with her husband, Gary, a medical doctor. She had been a student in one of my acute homeopathic prescribing courses and since then,

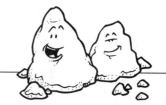

Natural Nuggets

People who are stressed have impaired healing. A study done by Kiecolt-Glaser and his colleagues compared 13 people caring for Alzheimer's patients to 13 subjects with similar ages and incomes. All subjects agreed to have a small wound made in their forearms. The caregivers took 49 days to heal while the control group took 39 days. It is well known that stress hormones retard the body's repairing mechanism.

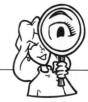

Curious Clues

Hypericum Perforatum is the Latin name for the popular plant St. John's Wort. The herbal form is used for anxiety, depression, as well as trauma and inflammations of the skin. Homeopathically, the diluted plant is used most for injuries affecting the nerves and spine. Sharp shooting pains make you think of Hypericum with injuries to the fingertips, head trauma, or fractures and sprains with shooting nerve-like pain.

she always carried her remedy kit with her. Luckily she had it on the ski slopes, because Gary had caught his finger on the binding of his ski and torn his fingernail half off. It hurt! While he was busy packing ice on the wound, Carol ran to get her kit. She remembered that Hypericum (better known as St. John's Wort) was the main remedy for nerve pain, particularly on the very sensitive fingertips and the tailbone. She administered to Gary a 30c dose under the tongue. Gary's pain vanished. The next time I saw Gary he recounted the story and admitted that he had never seen anything in his medical world like this! He was astonished that the pain could disappear within seconds of the pellets touching his tongue.

Nerve pain from injury or dental work may respond well to Hypericum Perforatum, the homeopathic form of St. John's Wort. It's particularly useful with injuries characterized by sharp shooting pain of the nerves or spine.

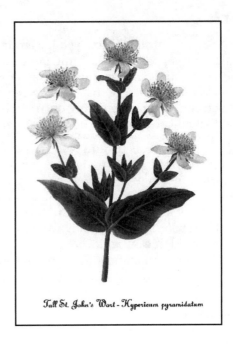

Tall St. John's Wort - *Hypericum pyramidatum*

The Least You Need to Know

➤ Many mild-to-moderate home emergencies can be safely and effectively treated with homeopathic medicines, while more severe traumas require homeopathy to be part of a comprehensive treatment plan.

➤ Apis, the highly diluted venom of a bumblebee, can be used to alleviate many insect stings and bites.

➤ For the best results in homeopathic emergency care, it's important to understand the total picture of the person, just as in chronic conditions.

➤ Most food poisoning is caused by bacteria that have been allowed to grow in foods and drinks.

➤ Homeopathic remedies such as Bryonia Album can help your body recover from the effects of the flu.

➤ Cantharis is useful for first-degree burns with or without blisters with burning pain relieved by cold.

➤ The homeopathic form of St. John's Wort (Hypericum) is often used for nerve-like pain resulting from traumas or inflammations of the skin.

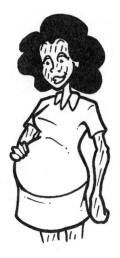

Chapter 14

Motherly Advice

In This Chapter

➤ Homeopathic help for infertility

➤ Get lasting relief from morning sickness with homeopathic remedies

➤ Lose labor pains with diluted solutions

➤ Discover relief from postpartum depression

➤ Manage mastitis safely for you and your baby with homeopathic medicines

---

Choosing to have a baby starts you on a journey where the course is not always clear or charted. This chapter is designed to help you meet challenges, both expected and unexpected, that may arise on your journey.

I'll start at the beginning, with infertility issues and all the intense emotions that surface, challenging you before you've even begun. I'll show you how to handle morning sickness and labor pains with homeopathic assistance. Postpartum depression and mastitis are conditions that also can be alleviated by homeopathic remedies.

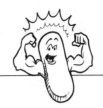

Potent Pellets

Women who are diagnosed with endometriosis (a condition when part of the uterine lining implants elsewhere in the abdominal cavity outside of the uterus), may be unable to conceive because of a missing protein. Alpha-beta 3 and leukemia inhibitory factor (LIF) play a crucial role in the embryo attaching to the uterus. Low levels of these proteins may explain the infertility rate among endometriosis patients.

Source: Fertility and Sterility, July 2000

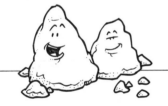

Natural Nuggets

Fertilization has to happen in the first third of the egg's journey; thus, the sperm and the egg must meet at the outer edge of the fallopian tube. The egg is ripe for fertilization for only about one day, and some experts believe it's for as little as eight hours.

Infertility: Intimacy by the Clock and the Calendar

Between 10 percent and 15 percent of all couples attempting their first pregnancy are unable to conceive. The disappointment, frustration, and sadness can be overwhelming at times. According to the National Institute of Child Health and Human Development, one year of unproductive, unprotected sexual intercourse is the standard definition for infertility. According to the Division of Urology at the University of North Carolina Medical School, apart from unexplainable reasons, 30 percent of the cases of infertile couples can be attributed solely to the man through low-sperm count or motility. Another 20 percent are abnormalities in both partners; the other 50 percent has to do with the physiology of the female.

A woman's fertility peaks at age 25 and continues to decline until menopause. Getting pregnant is not as easy as it may seem. It is an intricate process that is connected to a woman's hormonal system, metabolism, immune system, insulin regulation, and circulation. A healthy woman in her mid-20s has only a 20 percent to 30 percent chance of getting pregnant in any one month.

A girl is born with all the eggs she'll ever need. They are released throughout her reproductive years during a complex choreography of hormonal releases timed at ovulation, one egg per month at around day 14 of a 28-day cycle. The egg is swept through fallopian tubes to a waiting uterine lining that has been built up during the month to help the egg grow once it has been fertilized by the male sperm. Couples are encouraged to have intercourse one day before and one day after ovulation; the taking of basal thermometer (under the armpit) or home urine ovulation kits can predict the best time to try for a baby. If you can get past all the planning, studies show that a woman's enjoyment of intercourse increases lubrication of the vagina, and the contraction during orgasm helps propel the sperm along.

While there are many new medications and procedures for infertility treatments, couples often complain of physical discomfort and financial hardship. Homeopathic treatments are another option and may be a suitable solution worth trying.

Infertility (Presented by Savitri Clarke)

Jill and her husband have been trying for more than a year to have a baby. They are both young and healthy. All the medical tests were negative. Their doctor told them to see a specialist but instead they decided to try homeopathic treatment.

I asked if there had ever been anything remarkable about Jill's menstrual cycle. "I had a couple of cysts on my ovaries with my period, which burst on their own and went away." In a case with few physical symptoms, the nature of the person will be even more important than usual in leading to the correct remedy. I asked Jill to describe her nature. "I am a quiet, shy person. I don't like yelling and I don't yell unless I get really mad. I cry a lot though, all the time. I enjoy crying, cry in spurts and can cry anywhere. I don't like to confront people. I like to make people happy. I am very sensitive to rudeness. I have very high expectations of people. I would never tell them they hurt my feelings."

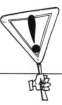

Caution Keeper

Kick the nicotine and caffeine habits for better fertility. Smokers are 30 percent less fertile than nonsmokers. Caffeine is related to delayed conception or infertility; just three cups of caffeinated beverages a day reduce your fertility by 28 percent.

Source: Natural Pregnancy, *Dr. Carrolle Jean-Murat, National Institutes of Health*

"I am very neat and organized, a perfectionist. It is hard for me to say no. I can't clean half the house or do just half the laundry."

"Maybe I am not going to be a good parent and God is sparing this child. My mother says we are too selfish and that is why. I have a lot of guilt. My mother is very dominating. I almost never yell back at her. When I am angry and I don't let it out, I grind my teeth at night."

When I analyzed Jill's case it was clear she was very sensitive, cried easily, and wanted to please. She suppressed her own feelings for what she thought was the good of others. Her high standards for herself and everyone around her made it hard for her to relax. The remedy I chose for Jill was Carcinosin.

Carcinosin is a nosode (a remedy made from human tissue or discharge) that comes from cancerous breast tissue. Like all remedies it is serially diluted so that there is no actual substance left, but the energetic properties of the remedy remain.

This remedy is useful for the following symptoms:

➤ Perfectionist, overly conscientious
➤ Sensitivity to rudeness, anger

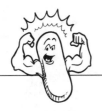

Potent Pellets

Science finally confirms what pregnant women have said for years: Smells trigger nausea during pregnancy. Levels of the female hormone estrogen, which naturally rise during a healthy pregnancy, also cause a heightened sense of smell.

Source: Nausea and Vomiting, Dr. Leroy Heinrich

➤ Tendency to suppress emotions, especially anger

➤ History of being dominated, often by an overbearing parent

➤ Great sensitivity to reprimand, disappointing others

➤ Need to push to the utmost of one's capacity, stretch oneself as far as possible

➤ Sympathetic

➤ Anxiety about family members

In addition, when questioned about dreams, Jill often dreamed about relatives who had died but were alive in the dream. It was as if they were actually communicating with her. People who need Carcinosin often are open to the spirit world and prophetic dreams are common.

Jill became pregnant within four months of taking the remedy. She had a healthy baby boy and returned a couple of years later for some homeopathic help with having a second child. The second time she conceived one month after the remedy and now has two lovely sons.

Morning Sickness: Slowing the Throwing

You're excited about being pregnant, thinking of all the little clothes and shoes you'll dress your little bundle of joy in when suddenly the bottom falls out of your stomach. Meals don't stay down and weakness is becoming a constant companion. You've become part of the 50 percent of all pregnant women who will experience morning sickness to some degree between weeks 6 and 12 of your first trimester. One out of 200 women will experience continuous nausea and vomiting that can result in dehydration, malnutrition, and unwanted weight loss.

Morning sickness nausea is often worse on an empty stomach. Try eating small, frequent meals throughout the day instead of the traditional big three. Bland starches such as breads, rice, and pasta digest quickly and are often better choices. Drinking plenty of fluids is important to prevent dehydration. A fetus's nutritional needs are minimal at first, but fluids are important to maintain. Midwives believe that lying down as often as possible, even without sleeping, is very helpful as it increases prolactin levels, which decreases nausea.

Homeopathics are safe, nontoxic, and nonhabit-forming treatments that can be used before, during, and after your baby is born.

Pregnancy-Induced Nausea and Vomiting

June was 6½ weeks pregnant when she came into my office tired, weak, and at the end of her rope. This was her second pregnancy, and she couldn't understand "why this one was going all wrong." She had the flu for several weeks at the beginning of her pregnancy and was still feeling tired and weak. Following the flu, she developed almost continuous indigestion, gas, and belching. Morning sickness followed. She did not want to eat, food did not appeal to her, and when she did eat, the result was heartburn. "This is so different from my first pregnancy. I'm sick of it already! Will I ever feel better?" She was cold but felt stuffy if she put extra clothes on; the heat made her nausea worse. She was becoming more irritable to her husband, saying things that hurt his feelings. She was hardly able to care for her daughter due to the heavy fatigue that consumed her. She was worrying more about the rest of her pregnancy.

I gave June Carbo Vegatabilis, the homeopathic remedy diluted from vegetable charcoal.

Within a week, June was feeling less fatigued, with lower levels of nausea. Her vomiting decreased rapidly over the next week to negligible amounts. Her energy returned, and the multiple gastro-distress disappeared. She regained her happy grin and disposition and carried full term to a normal delivery.

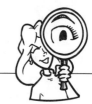

Curious Clues

Carbo Vegatabilis shares some keynote symptoms with June's complaints. These helped me arrive at this remedy choice:

➤ Morning sickness

➤ Serious indigestion and burping

➤ Increased intestinal gas

➤ Heartburn

➤ Great fatigue

➤ Cold, but no desire to be covered

➤ Increased irritability, harsh remarks often directed at the family

Labor Pains: No Pain, All Gain

Many women I've met are excited about bringing their new baby home, but they are more nervous about the experience of giving birth. Although the apprehension concerning what's about to happen can still be high, birthing classes may help to answer questions and concerns.

Many obstetric units use labor, delivery, and postpartum rooms so that you are with support people in a comfortable, friendly environment. A growing number of women want to be as comfortable as possible during their delivery, but are concerned about the anesthesia and pudendal blocks that may be used. Homeopathic medicines offer sound nonchemical solutions that can be satisfying and effective when prescribed properly.

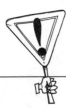

Caution Keeper

Premature or preterm labor means going into labor or breaking water before 37 weeks of pregnancy. One in 10 babies are born prematurely in the United States. Four out of five women in premature labor arrive at the hospital too late for treatment—three out of four premature babies die. Call your health provider if any unusual signs of labor are present three weeks or more before your due date.

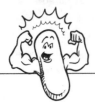

Potent Pellets

Women who have long and stressful labors or who are giving birth for the first time often take longer to lactate. A study suggests lactation consultants would be beneficial.

Source: American Journal of Clinical Nutrition, *August 2000*

Labor and Delivery (Presented by Pamela J. Herring)

My daughter Sarah was a few days overdue for her fourth baby. She called me, as her mom and a homeopathic doctor, about 10 P.M. to say she was in severe pain and was leaving for the hospital. I suggested that she take out the birthing kit that I had given her and asked her to describe her symptoms for a remedy. The pains, she said, were in the lower back and were severe. She had to walk around because of restlessness.

We gave her a dose of 30c of Coffea and told her to come over to our house since we lived five minutes from the hospital. When she and her husband, Tom, arrived, she said the remedy worked like magic. We sent Tom to bed as he would be coaching her later at the birthing room in the hospital, and Sarah settled on the couch while I helped her with the labor through the night. She took repeated doses of Coffea whenever the pain got severe and it would dissipate it. By 6 A.M. the contractions were close together so we woke up Tom and sent them to the hospital while my husband and I stayed at home with their other two children. About three hours later Sarah called to say the doctor insisted on giving her a prescription painkiller and subsequently the labor stopped completely. They then wanted to induce labor, which prompted Sarah's call. I told her to take out her trusty kit again and take one dose of Cimicifuga 200c. She took it and within a minute or two the contractions started again. Forty-five minutes later she gave birth to a healthy seven-pound girl, Isabella Rose.

Cimicifuga is also a remedy for overdue labor. It is one of the main remedies for stalled contractions. There are dozens of rubrics of Cimicifuga pertaining to labor.

Homeopathy spared Sarah several interventions during labor. She definitely did not want to suffer the effects of a drug-induced labor, but preferred the gentle, safe and effective experience of a homeopathic remedy.

Breast Infections: A Mastitis Moment

Incomplete emptying of the milk ducts or a tight bra can cause a plugged duct in your breast. If this is not resolved, mastitis can occur. A baby's strong sucking may cause tiny cracks in the skin of your nipple, which allows bacteria to enter and be nourished by the sweet breast milk, also causing a breast infection. Mastitis affects about 2 percent of nursing mothers who experience the symptoms of a hard, sore area usually on one breast, redness, swelling and pain on the area, fever (mild or high), chills, aches, and a general feeling of being ill.

Your health-care provider may suggest antibiotics. Other recommendations include drinking plenty of fluids, getting plenty of rest, and applying moist heat with a hot water bottle and moist washcloth. Continue nursing your baby or the ducts will remain full and overfill, which can worsen the condition. As you will see in the next patient's story, homeopathic options can be a safe and reliable choice for both mother and baby.

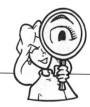

Curious Clues

Based upon Sarah's symptoms, I decided to prescribe Coffea, the homeopathic diluted from coffee. This remedy was indicated by the following rubrics that are looked up in a homeopathic repertory (see Chapter 8, "Your First Visit to a Homeopath") to assist you in finding the best choice:

➤ Back pain during delivery

➤ Back pain, lumbar region

➤ Back pain excessive during labor

➤ Physical restlessness

Acute Mastitis (Presented by Savitri Clarke)

Mary was a happy new mother with a lovely robust four-month old little boy. She was enjoying breastfeeding her son and their bond was growing stronger and stronger. One morning she began experiencing pain in her right breast, which got even worse when the baby nursed. A hard swelling was forming on her breast that was red and sensitive to touch. "Please tell me what to do. I feel very strongly that I don't want to take antibiotics while I am nursing my baby." Her symptoms sounded like a clogged milk duct and as she had no other symptoms, it was recommended that she use hot moist compresses on the breast, try to rest and stay reclining as much as possible, and have the baby nurse as much as possible. If her condition was not improving in a few hours, she should come into the office.

She arrived very shaken and upset a few hours later. "The lump was getting harder and darker red, almost purple, and the pain was getting worse and would spread through my whole body when he nursed. On the way here I started getting severe chills. The only thing that helps the pain is to press on my breast with my hand. I feel very spacey, almost dizzy." Mary indeed had a 102°F fever that had come on in a matter of minutes. Examination revealed a hard reddish-purple lump on her right breast. With these systemic symptoms it was crucial that Mary got a fast-acting effective remedy or began antibiotics very soon. Mary was given the remedy Phytolacca.

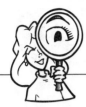

Curious Clues

Mary was given one dose of homeopathic poke root, called Phytolacca. Phytolacca was chosen because ...

➤ It has an affinity for the female glandular system.

➤ Inflammation of breast, mastitis.

➤ Swellings, especially of the breast, usually if purple in color.

➤ The pain is relieved by pressing with the hand.

I had Mary stay in the waiting room because, given the acute nature of her symptoms, if my remedy choice was correct she should experience relief in a short period of time. Within 15 minutes her chills started to disappear, the lump began to soften, the pain lessened, and her mental clarity returned. She returned home with some extra doses of the remedy in case the lump and pain returned. Mary called the next day to say, "I feel fine now! I can't believe how quickly the remedy worked." She had not needed to repeat the remedy and was grateful that she was able to avoid antibiotics.

Postpartum Depression (PPD): Despair Out of Nowhere

After all the rigors of carrying a child and birthing your baby into the world, it doesn't seem fair that you may experience despair about 24 hours after delivery. Between 50 percent and 80 percent of women will experience postpartum blues for up to two weeks following the birth of their baby. Reassurance and assistance with the increased household duties is usually the only recommended treatment. Approximately 10 percent to 20 percent of new mothers will go on to a deeper, more disturbing postpartum depression between two and eight weeks after giving birth.

Many women, especially nursing mothers, are reluctant to take antidepressants, since all medications are absorbed in the breast milk. Zoloft, Paxil, and tricyclics are short-acting serotonin neuro-uptake inhibitors and are frequently prescribed because they accumulate at lower levels in an infant's blood and do not appear to produce changes in cognitive development. Many mothers are opting to use homeopathic medicines that are safe to use while nursing, and when properly used, can effectively help you during this period of depression and unrest. For an example of homeopathic whole healing, take a look at the next patient's story.

Postpartum Depression (Presented by Savitri Clarke)

Nancy, a long-time patient of mine, called, desperate to see me. "I just had my first baby and I feel like I am flipping out. I just don't know if I can do it. I need help." She arrived a few days later with a two-month-old baby in tow. She looked worried and exhausted.

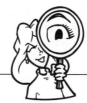

Curious Clues

There are many possible symptoms of postpartum depression (PPD), including ...

➤ Insomnia or prolonged sleep, even when the baby is awake.

➤ Extreme concern over the baby or lack of interest and no feelings.

➤ Feeling unable to love the baby or family.

➤ Panic attacks.

➤ Sadness, excessive crying.

➤ Feelings of doubt, guilt, or hopelessness.

➤ Frequent calls to the pediatrician with an inability to be reassured.

➤ Thoughts of death or suicide.

She responded with almost a startle to every movement or sound the baby made. It was as if she were constantly afraid she would neglect something or do the wrong thing. This resulted in an intense hypervigilance.

"The birth went great. Only nine hours altogether. I only pushed for a couple of hours and it wasn't that bad. The baby was fine. I had horrible back labor during the pushing and bad back pain after the birth. It was like a bad spasm. My back still hurts and my back and legs are still weak. I am breastfeeding my baby and now I am getting blocked ducts. My breasts get splotchy red and very painful. I had to consult a lactation consultant and use an electric pump. It was frustrating for me. Just one more thing I had to do, worry about her weight gain. I hadn't expected that to be an issue."

"Emotionally the first few weeks were terrible. I was angry and irritable, especially to my mother, who came the second week. I was impatient and very critical of her. I felt trapped upstairs and I cried a lot. When my mother went home I felt hurt and I am sure she did, too. I am so afraid I am going to do something wrong. I am having dreams about something happening to her or losing her because I wasn't paying close enough attention. The baby is crying in the dream, needing me. I have also had dreams about the police and feeling like I committed some horrible crime."

"I have joined a mom's group. All these women are talking to their babies. I get inse-cure about how much I should be stimulating her. I worry about what these other mothers think when they see me with her, or for that matter, even what you will think!"

Nancy was given the remedy homeopathic Bamboo (*Bambusa Arundinacae*).

Here are a few ideas that led me to choose the homeopathic medicine Bamboo:

➤ While bamboo can be bent, it can also be strong as iron, growing as much as a foot a day, and can grow through concrete or asphalt.

➤ This remedy type has a strong work ethic, especially when it comes to the family unit.

➤ They have tremendous anxiety about the family as evidenced in dreams of neg-lected children, lost children, and the police.

➤ They can get into a state of feeling overwhelmed where they have taken on a tremendous amount of work and then feel unequal to the task.

➤ They can then easily start feeling they are a failure.

➤ Very sensitive, weepy, and insecure, never knowing when the next catastrophe will befall them, yet they continue to try harder.

➤ Physically they often have back problems or a weakness in that area.

Nancy returned one month after receiving the remedy. She reported that she felt stronger, more secure in herself and in her abilities to mother her baby. "It doesn't seem so hard now. I don't care as much what others think but am relying on my own instincts now." She was even willing to ask for help from her husband, which had been hard for her before. Her anxiety was much decreased and her dreams had be-come more peaceful. In addition, she felt her back was getting stronger and was now experiencing very little pain.

I am in awe at the focus and multitasking that is required of a woman through the entire process of giving life to another. New mothers must learn a host of complex skills, while feeling a broad range of new emotions. Homeopathy can lend a helping hand so that your own dedication will handle the situation.

The next chapter will continue to deliver useful assistance for such conditions as PMS, painful periods, menopause, and chronic bladder infections.

The Least You Need to Know

➤ A healthy woman in her mid-20s has only a 20 percent to 30 percent chance of getting pregnant in any one month.

➤ Nicotine and caffeine decrease your odds of fertility.

➤ Fifty percent of all pregnant women will experience some form of morning sickness.

➤ Homeopathic remedies are safe to take before, during, and after your pregnancy for a host of ailments.

➤ Phytolacca (homeopathic poke root), when properly prescribed, can be an effective treatment for breast infections.

➤ Ten percent to twenty percent of new mothers will experience postpartum depression (PPD).

➤ Homeopathic remedies can be used to shake off the black cloud of postpartum depression.

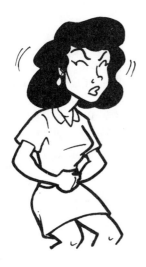

Chapter 15

Bummin' at the Plumbin'

In This Chapter

➤ Put an end to PMS with homeopathy

➤ Discover homeopathic ways to ease painful periods

➤ Manage menopause using homeopathic medicines

➤ Learn how homeopathics can curb bladder infections

➤ Treat chronic Candida with effective homeopathic treatments

---

Considerable anguish, frustration, and irritation has been related to me by my female patients when their specialized anatomy and monthly menstrual cycle are out of balance. I've witnessed highly motivated and accomplished women get stopped in their tracks when hormones derail their day as in PMS, painful periods, and menopause. Similarly, chronic bladder infections and Candida are painful and annoying reminders of female susceptibilities.

In a society that promotes an ability to function without pause or flaws, these conditions pose a potential obstacle. We're going to discuss these conditions, the homeopathic treatments available, and household tips that can make a lasting difference in the quality of your life.

Premenstrual Syndrome

Are you among the 70 percent to 75 percent of women who say they experience some form of *premenstrual syndrome* (or *PMS*) in their lifetime? If so, then one or two weeks before menstruation begins, you experience one or more of the typical symptoms such as weight gain, breast tenderness, abdominal bloating, backache, joint pain, acne, cramps, fatigue, insomnia, anxiety, food cravings, or personality changes.

Some women do not notice much of anything before their period, while an estimated 30 percent to 40 percent report daily activities being disrupted, and 5 percent of women say they become completely disabled by their PMS.

Cutting back or eliminating refined sugars, salt, red meat, junk foods, coffee, teas, and colas can help to reduce PMS. Try adding whole grains, legumes (beans, peas, lentils), and oils such as black currant, flaxseed, and evening primrose. Homeopathic treatment is a great complement to healthy living and eating. You've suffered long enough.

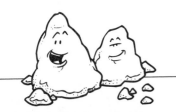

Dose of Info

A variation of **premenstrual syndrome** (or **PMS**) in which severe mood symptoms predominate is called premenstrual dysphoric disorder (PMDD). This condition is characterized by strong emotions that are triggered by the normal hormonal oscillations of the menstrual cycle.

Natural Nuggets

Eating a low-fat, vegetarian diet can reduce the severity and length of menstrual cramps and PMS. Researchers at the Georgetown University School of Medicine feel that a low-fat, no-animal-product diet minimizes the thickness of the built-up uterine wall, whose sloughing off triggers menstrual cramps.

PMS

About a week before my period starts, my psycho sister takes over my body," says Betty, who has come in for a homeopathic consult for PMS and psoriasis. "I normally feel okay to be with people, but before my period, I can cry so easily, get angry at my boyfriend, and just want to be alone. I don't want to be this way, but at this time, I can get cold-hearted and scream at my boyfriend."

Betty went on to say that stress at work was high. Normally she can get through it, but not during her PMS. She felt overwhelmed and "not with it." She went on to say that she was born with psoriasis 32 years ago and did not grow out of it as many of her doctors thought. She noticed her skin was worse from stress, sweat, and PMS. Lately her psoriasis was breaking out in bright red thick patches on the back of her head, elbows, hips, and knees. She often scratched until it bled, which only gave temporary relief. She was normally chilly but felt much colder before and during her menstrual cycle. She had problems with

PMS since she was a teenager, got on birth control pills, but came off because she didn't like the way she felt. She has tried topical creams including steroids for her psoriasis, thus far without relief.

I gave Betty Sepia, the diluted homeopathic remedy of cuttle fish or squid ink.

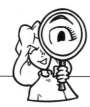

Curious Clues

Sepia is a well-known polycrest (meaning "having many uses") in homeopathy. It is versatile and can be easily found in most local homeopathic pharmacies. The physical symptoms of PMS narrowed my search for a remedy down to only about 200 choices! The combination of how she felt emotionally joined with the physical complaints led me to try Sepia. These are some of the criteria I used from her story:

➤ Crying, even without knowing why

➤ Cutting remarks followed by remorse

➤ Disconnected and indifferent to loved ones/family

➤ Irritable

➤ Premenstrual irritability and weepiness

➤ Desire to be alone, yet despises being completely alone

➤ Psoriasis with thick parchment-like skin

➤ Feeling overwhelmed and mentally sluggish

The following month, Betty told me her menstrual cycle was less eventful with fewer of the out-of-control emotions. Her psoriasis had no flare-ups despite her work being particularly stressful. In a three-month follow-up, Betty told me her "psycho sister" had not come to visit. She was sleeping better with no abnormal irritability, standoffishness, or disconnected feelings. She was no longer scratching her psoriasis at night, and her skin was overall feeling and looking much better. Six months later, she said, "I've reached a balanced phase. I'm not having any flare-ups with my skin and have cut out my creams and ointments. In the past with PMS, I'd get crazy, now I'm fine! I don't feel stressed out anymore; I'm much more mellow all the time." In checking with her about six months later, she was still fine and didn't need to repeat her remedy.

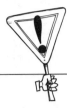

Caution Keeper

Chocolate is the most craved substance with 40 percent of women and 15 percent of men admitting to regular cravings. There are over 400 discrete compounds that have been identified in chocolate with many affecting how you feel. The sweet and fat combination may directly stimulate brain opiate receptors, the same cells that respond to heroin and morphine. The average American consumes 11.5 pounds of chocolate per year.

Source: onhealth.com

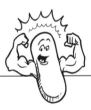

Potent Pellets

She has such different moods. One day she is all smiles and happiness. Other days, there is no living with her. Throughout a woman's life, waves of emotions mimic the sea, so often innocent and still, yet sometimes wild and turbulent.

Source: An Essay on Women, *Somonides, 6th century* B.C.E.

Painful Periods: Dealing with Dysmenorrhea

Pain and anxiety can be monthly markers when painful menstrual dysmenorrhea or periods occur. Primary dysmenorrhea is thought to result from uterine muscle contractions as sloughed-off tissue from the uterine walls attempts to pass through a narrow opening in the cervix. Lack of exercise and malpositioning of the uterus are thought to contribute to this monthly experience. Secondary dysmenorrhea is associated with conditions such as endometriosis and pelvic inflammatory disease.

Conventional medical treatments include applying local heat to the abdomen, drug therapy for pain, and corrective surgery with secondary dysmenorrhea. Homeopathy can offer a tremendous amount of help in making women's monthly cycles less stressful and traumatic. Read the next patient's story and see how a woman at her wit's end found help with homeopathic medicine.

Painful Periods (Presented by Savitri Clarke)

Maria is very excited when she calls for her appointment. "I sure hope she can help me. My periods are getting worse and worse. I hate taking the medicine the doctors give me and it barely helps anyway."

When Maria comes for her initial visit she begins talking before she even sits down. She is Italian, very animated, excited, with bright red cheeks. She begins. "Four years ago it started with bad headaches. I never had a problem before. I saw hundreds of gynecologists and they couldn't solve it. When I feel very bad I start sweating a lot and become extremely weak. I must lie down then or I fall, sometimes I faint. I feel terrible, like I am in labor almost. This lasts an hour and a half. There is nausea and throwing up, then I feel very cold and I shake. I need four or five blankets and I keep shaking. Finally it goes away." I asked her how her periods were when she first started getting them.

"When I was younger the pain was even worse. Once at work they took me to the emergency room. It comes on all of a sudden. I don't have the strength to talk. Violent retching, I just can't help it."

Maria's husband is reluctant to spend money on homeopathy but Maria is desperate. "We argue about money. I want to go to Italy, and he doesn't allow me to do it so we argue. Then I start going away from him and feel like I want to get divorced. I have a very hard head. When I want to do something nobody stops me. But he does. He won't let me spend the money. What I have to go through!" She stands up as she is talking, gesticulates strongly, and gets very worked up. "How can he do this to me? How can he tell me I can't go?"

Maria worries a lot about her children. She dreams about something happening to her children. She also used to dream cats were jumping on top of her and scratching her.

I gave Maria Lac Lioninum, homeopathic lion's milk. Maria's headaches and menstrual symptoms greatly reduced within two months of taking the remedy. Over the last two years, she is almost pain free and has had virtually none of those intense episodes she initially described. She sings praises to homeopathy!

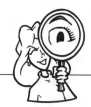

Curious Clues

Maria's issue is one of not wanting anyone to dominate her. That combined with the feeling of desperation, the anxiety about her children, and the dreams of cats scratching her led me to the remedy Lac Lioninum (lion's milk). People who need animal remedies tend to have strong issues around basic survival. Maria cannot tolerate her husband ruling over her. This is the feeling of the lion.

Menopause: The Range of "The Change"

The "Big M" and "The Change" were code words for *menopause* that our mothers and grandmothers used to whisper, referring to a natural transition in a woman's life called menopause. Fortunately, women and men are reading, learning, and discussing a normal change that occurs in a woman's life sometime between 45 and 55. While 51 is an average age for women to stop ovulating and menstruating (menopause), pre- or *perimenopause* lasts about 5 to 10 years before the last menstrual period.

Each woman's experience of menopause is individual, ranging from barely noticeable, to the common perimenopausal experiences as irregular

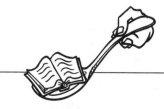

Dose of Info

Menopause is when your fertility comes to an end; **perimenopause** is the transition marked by symptoms that show the decline in your body's ovary production of the reproductive hormones estrogen and progesterone.

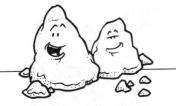

Natural Nuggets

Confused about the menopausal maze? Try contacting the North American Menopause Society at PO Box 94527, Cleveland, OH 44101-4527 (440-442-7550). They can send you a "MenoPak," which includes a menopause guidebook, a list of discussion groups, and menopause specialists in your area.

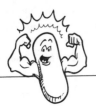

Potent Pellets

Some herbal extracts have strong estrogenic properties. Researchers have emained dong qui, vitex, Chinese ginseng, American ginseng, black cohosh, red raspberry leaf, blue cohosh, licorice root, squaw vine, milk thistle seeds, hops, and wild yam root. They may be useful for women who prefer to take these as a subsitute for pharmaceutical medications. Always advise your homeopath if you are taking any of these herbs.

Source: Veterans Affairs Medical Center, University of Pittsburgh, Pennsylvania

menstrual periods, hot flashes, vaginal dryness and itching, diminished sex drive, difficulty sleeping, mood swings, depression, and anxiety.

Meet the estrogen family whose members rise and fall over the course of a woman's cycle:

➤ **Estradial:** Dominant from puberty to menopause, originates in the ovaries and adrenal glands.

➤ **Estrone:** Dominant after menopause, originates from fat cells and the liver.

➤ **Estriol:** Dominant during pregnancy, originates from the placenta during pregnancy and the liver.

Source: Estrogen Dilemmas, *Dr. Laura Pawlak*

Diminishing estrogen can put you at risk for cardiovascular disease, osteoporosis, and vaginal atrophy. Hormone replacement therapy (HRT) is often recommended by conventional medicine. Learn the facts and your own risk factors before beginning HRT.

Many women are living a third of their lives after menopause. I suggest getting educated about options that will have an impact for many years to come. There may be a period of disbelief and frustration that your body is not the same as it's always been, but careful planning with consistent follow-through with healthy foods, exercise, and yes, homeopathy, can cut down on the challenges and help bring you into your full power and wisdom at this stage of your life.

Perimenopause

"I'm want my old body back," said Janine, a 48-year-old hard-working mother and office manager of a family business. "We've been busting our butts, are doing okay, finally want to take a break and all this happens." Janine complained of hot flashes, fatigue, poor sleep, restlessness, and anxiety. She was borderline anemic despite a good diet, felt cold most of the time, and only liked hot flashes because they initially warmed her up before she overheated. She'd spent her life at home juggling raising a family and the growing demand of a family business. She worried about her kids, and she worried about the business all day long. At night, she'd get ideas that would rattle around in her mind, most often little things that could be taken care of easily. These thoughts plus her hot flashes got worse at night, and she could often be found pacing around her home office at night or flipping through late-night TV. She normally liked to exercise, but since perimenopause she got exhausted much easier. She was becoming more "touchy" and anxious, often being startled by noises in the house and could not stand to have her nerves rattled by loud music or television noises. I gave Janine the remedy Ferrum Arsenicosum.

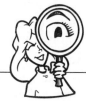

Curious Clues

What do you get when you combine highly diluted homeopathic ferrum (iron) and arsenic? For Janine, it was homeopathic help for perimenopausal symptoms. Have you picked out a few of the important points of her case? My reasons for giving this remedy include ...

➤ Hot flashes.

➤ Fatigue, anemia.

➤ Anxiety and restlessness, worse at night.

➤ Worrying about insignificant things.

➤ Feeling cold.

➤ Sensitivity to music.

➤ Working hard and pushing through tasks.

➤ Highly organized (a metal group symptom).

➤ Extreme dedication and worry about work and family tasks.

Janine began to feel better with her hot flashes in about one week. On her six-week follow-up appointment, she noticed her anxiety level was lower. She was still concerned about her kids and their business, but her behavior was more appropriate. Her sleeping patterns were better and naturally her general energy improved. She has used this remedy intermittently for two years, often going months without a single dose.

Bladder Infections

Bladder infections, also known as cystitis, are one of the most common conditions among women of all ages. According to a new study at the University of Washington School of Medicine, an estimated seven million episodes of acute cystitis occur annually in the United States with an annual cost of $1 billion. The study further showed the term "honeymoon cystitis" is still accurate in that having sexual intercourse increased the risk of developing the condition. *Escherichia coli* (*E. coli*) bacteria found in fecal material is responsible for up to 90 percent of all urinary tract infections (UTI). Fecal-contaminated bacteria gains access to the bladder through the urethra.

Women are 30 times more likely to have cystitis than men due mostly to the different lengths of the urethra (women's urethras are just 1½ inches long, while men have urethras about 8 inches long). Men experience UTIs with obstructions like urinary stones or enlarged prostate. According to the National Bladder Foundation, an estimated 3 percent of girls and 1 percent of boys have UTIs by the age of 11. Among elderly women living in nursing homes or hospitalized, 20 percent to 50 percent will develop asymptomatic bacteriuria, which is a UTI without symptoms. The elderly and pregnant women are at risk for this type of UTI, which is symptom free but can still develop into serious infections of the kidneys if left untreated.

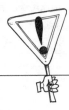

Caution Keeper

The U.S. Census Bureau estimates that there will be a 12 percent increase in the number of bladder diseases over the next 15 years, with a dramatic 28 percent increase among women and men 40 to 59 years of age.

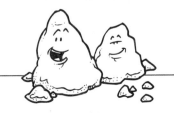

Natural Nuggets

Drinking cranberry juice to prevent a UTI really does work! Researchers have recently found that cranberries and blueberries contain infection-fighting compounds called tannins. A 10-ounce glass of cranberry juice helps prevent bacteria from attaching to the urinary tract.

Source: The New England Journal of Medicine, October 8, 2000

Chronic Urinary Tract Infections

"I worry about it all the time. I get burning after urination, cramping pains, and I can't go 20 minutes without having to go to the bathroom." Alisha had been given a diagnosis of chronic cystitis or bladder infection, but had a urologist who also thought she exhibited symptoms of interstitial cystitis, a more serious bladder condition. Alisha was nervous about many things and had been since she was a little girl. She stated that she covers it well by being witty and clever. At our visits, she would come close to doing a comedy routine. At one point, she confided to me that she had been demoralized as a teenager. "My mother divorced when I was 13 years old. She was an alcoholic. I never knew what I'd find when I got home. Mom was usually passed out on the couch, and when she tried to cook, she'd start a grease fire." Alisha paused for several seconds, began to tear up, and said that her mom's friends had been bad to her in a lot of ways. She had been unable to get mad as a kid and felt sad and anxious. She then moved on to a joke about how she breaks up with boyfriends quickly before they can break up with her. She likes to have the man take over, but gets scared, breaks up with them, and feels lonely afterward.

I prescribed the homeopathic form of the cockle Xanthium Spinosum.

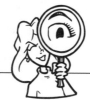

Curious Clues

At first I gave Alisha Staphysagnia, a remedy that has many of the same important components of urinary tract conditions with a history of abusive situations. This did not work well. I went on to look at Xanthium Spinosum, because it reflects the long-time anger and humiliation that is masked by humor and often presents as anxiety. Other findings that would indicate this remedy include ...

➤ Reoccurring bladder infections or intestinal cystitis.

➤ Abusive, tormenting situations, especially sexual.

➤ Open, witty, animated jokesters.

➤ Choosing relationships where they are dominated by the partner.

➤ Anxiety.

The first few months following the remedy Alisha had a resolution of most of her urinary condition. She still had some discomfort following sexual arousal; however, it did not lead to a full inflammation as she previously experienced. She had a gradual lessening of her general anxiety. It took almost a year for her to get into a healthy relationship, lose most of her anxiety, and begin to trust again. Healing this long-term anxiety was helped by homeopathy, her therapist, and the willingness of Alisha to actively face and confront the obstacles to her happiness. I saw her about two years later. She had not needed to take the remedy, was still a witty person, but no longer used humor to cover up her anxiety. No bladder discomfort was reported.

The homeopathic remedy Xanthium Spinosum is made from the highly diluted form of the cockle. This remedy is useful for witty persons suffering from chronic bladder infections, anxiety, fears, and most often a history of abuse.

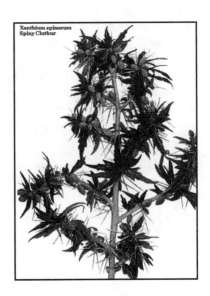

Xanthium spinosum
Spiny Clutbur

Candida: The Beast of the Yeast

Candida infections account for about 80 percent of all major systemic fungal infections. According to the *Merck Manual* (1999), it is now the fourth most common organism found in bloodstream infections and is the most prevalent cause of fungal infections in immune-compromised people such as advanced cancer or AIDS patients. Candida infections rose fivefold during the 1980s, making it one of the most common hospital-acquired infections and responsible for prolonged hospitalizations.

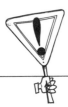

Caution Keeper

Oral thrush in an infant looks like white spots that may resemble milk spots and form a thick coating on the tongue and gums. Thrush can spread from the baby to the mother's nipples in breastfeeding and can lead to a situation where mother and baby continually reinfect each other. Check with your health-care provider if you suspect this is happening.

Candida albicans is a common parasitic yeastlike fungus that naturally inhabits our intestines, genital tract, mouth, throat, and esophagus. There is usually a healthy balance between this fungus and other naturally occurring bacteria in our bodies, but when something occurs to weaken our immune system, the fungi are allowed to multiply, causing an infection known as candidiasis. The fungus can then travel through the bloodstream to many parts of the body.

Treatments of Candida infection with conventional medicine are typically given through antifungal medications such as Fluconazole, Amphotericin B, depending on the strain of Candida that has been identified, or if you have developed fluconazole-resistant organisms from continued use. I have found that homeopathy and nutritional changes can break the pattern of chronic Candida infections. Your immune system is strengthened, and the normal checks and balances of your body are restored.

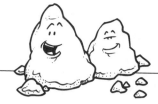

Natural Nuggets

Nutrition is an important part of ending the cycle of chronic Candida. Some ideas to consider include ...

➤ Take supplemental acidophilus and bifidus, naturally occurring bacteria for the bowels and vagina.

➤ Cut out sugar, fruit juices, yeasts, and products made from these ingredients; they feed the Candida fungus.

➤ Eat vegetables, fish, and gluten-free grains such as brown rice and millet.

➤ Drink distilled water only.

➤ Avoid aged cheeses, alcohol, baked goods, chocolate, dried fruits, fermented foods, all grains that contain gluten, ham, honey, potatoes, raw mushrooms, and vinegar.

Chronic Candida (Presented by Savitri Clarke)

Tricia came to me for help with chronic Candida (yeast). She had been "feeling more on the fragile side of things." She describes herself as "not sickly, always able to go to work, never bedridden, but not well."

When asked about her Candida symptoms she described "a hungover feeling in the morning. My stomach is anxious, stressed, gaseous. I break out on the chest and back with a rash. It is dry and bumpy, gets worse in the winter and is much worse at night. I have had the rash for three years. I don't feel free. I have to always wear clothes that will cover it up." She is embarrassed to tell me that her stools have a very foul odor making her reluctant to use a public rest room. "How can I get rid of the smell for the next person?"

Tricia gets migraine headaches and has very painful, sharp ovary pains with her periods. She has recurrent vaginal yeast infections that she treated with Monistat. She has

177

had a history of abnormal pap smears with one cryosurgery treatment for cervical dysplasia. She has very frequent urination, often 10 times by early afternoon.

When I ask Tricia to describe her nature she says, "I tend to be gentle, not wild, overly mannered sometimes. I grew up with a sister that was beautiful with long blonde hair. I had short hair and was confused for a boy a lot as a kid. It is an image I have grown up with: Am I a boy or a girl? I can still feel that although my essence is feminine I don't have that female thing."

Tricia's work involves frequent presentations to groups. "I don't want to step out into the world without the loveliness of clothes and the color that makeup can add. I admire people that are natural but I can't do that."

"Adolescence was traumatic for me. My skin started to change with acne. It was traumatic for my mother, too. She got me into makeup really young, terrible thick makeup. I have memories of not doing a good job. My sister said she hated riding the bus with me I was so made up." I gave Tricia the homeopathic remedy Thuja.

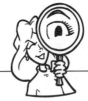

Curious Clues

Tricia had a history of pleasing other people. She grew up unsure of her femininity and learned from her mother to hide her flaws and weaknesses. She had the feeling there was something bad or wrong in her that she always needed to cover up. The remedy chosen for Tricia was Thuja, homeopathic red cedar. People needing this remedy often describe a confusion of identity, a feeling of fragility (as if they are made of glass), and the need to cover up that, which is not attractive to others. Thuja is a major remedy for chronic yeast infections, ovary pains with the period, headaches, blurred vision, and frequent daytime urination.

Tricia returned six weeks later, saying, "I am doing really great. I feel like you gave me a jump start, a jolt. There are a lot of changes going on. It all feels like this great spiraling upward. Initially, I had a few days of headaches but then I started to feel much better. The dry, red bumpy rash is gone. I don't feel as fragile. I have been feeling expansive at work; I was stuck before and now I can finally make the changes I need to make."

Tricia continued to improve needing only one more dose of Thuja nine months later.

The Least You Need to Know

➤ Cutting back on sugars, salt, red meat, junk foods, coffee, teas, and colas can help to reduce PMS.

➤ Properly given homeopathic medicines can safely treat PMS, painful periods, and perimenopausal symptoms.

➤ Many women are living a third of their lives after menopause; homeopathy combined with good nutrition and consistent exercise can help make these years healthy.

➤ Xanthium Spinosum is helpful for individuals with chronic bladder infections and a history of anxiety and abuse.

➤ Eighty percent of all major systemic fungal infections are caused by Candida; proper nutrition and homeopathy can restore the normal balance of the bacteria.

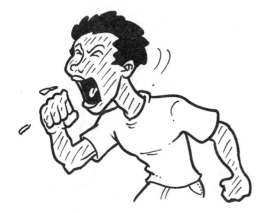

Chapter 16

The Respiration Station

> **In This Chapter**
>
> ➤ Breathe easier with homeopathic relief
>
> ➤ Discover how homeopaths soothe your sore throat and comfort your cough
>
> ➤ Ease your wheeze from asthma by using time-tested homeopathic remedies
>
> ➤ Wave bye-bye to the pain and suffering of chronic sinusitis
>
> ➤ Allergy symptoms disappear using homeopathic principles and treatments

In this chapter, we deal with common bronchial ailments such as coughs, sore throats, and asthma. You'll also learn how homeopathy can help with bothersome allergies and chronic sinusitis.

Sore Throat: Pain in the Pipeline

Pain, soreness, rawness, and burning in your throat are all common signs of a sore throat. We experience sore throats all through our lives. They are usually caused by viral infections such as in a common cold or bacterial infections like *Streptococcus pyogenes,* or "strep." Other sources of throat irritation include extremely hot foods or drinks, the old pizza burn, fumes, smoke, or dust.

Most acute sore throats resolve themselves within a few days or a week. Chronic sore throats may signal more concern to rule out mononucleosis, Epstein-Barr virus, *Herpes simplex,* or measles and chicken pox in children. Antibiotics are commonly prescribed.

A visit with your primary care provider will settle any questions regarding the origin of your sore throat. Many parents and concerned adults have been using homeopaths to deal with the symptoms of pain and swelling, while simultaneously strengthening the immune system. This is particularly necessary if the origin of your pain is viral and antibiotics will have no effect. Check out the options one mother used to help her child in the next patient's story.

Pediatric Sore Throat (Presented by Savitri Clarke)

Jane brought in her 17-month-old daughter, Sandra, after a diagnosis of acute viral tonsillitis. Her medical doctor had assured her that antibiotics wouldn't help in Sandra's case. Her fever was over 103°F when she was first diagnosed. Now, two days later, she ran an almost constant 100°F fever. The child was miserable: whining, complaining, and needing to be held constantly. Her tonsils were enormous with much pus exuding from them. Sandra was barely eating or drinking, presumably because of the pain in her throat. She shrieked a lot with the pain, and woke up screaming from every nap. Her mood was irritable and capricious—she would really want something only to cast it aside when she was given it. There was no pleasing her. Jane said she had never been inconsolable like this before and that it was very difficult to deal with her.

When I asked about her nature before the illness Jane described Sandra as bossy and fairly fearless. She loves to clean up and is unhappy going down for a nap if all her toys aren't picked up first.

Ideally, the remedy that would help Sandra should cover her acute symptoms but also fit her general nature. She was given the remedy Chamomilla.

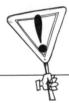

Caution Keeper

"Strep" (*Streptococcus pyogenes*) can live in your throat and nose for months without causing any harm. About 18 percent of healthy people have the strep bug living uneventfully in their mouth and nose. If you've been under stress and your immune system takes a dive, you could develop the characteristic sore throat, fever, white pus on tonsils, and tender lymph nodes in the neck. Untreated, the condition can lead to severe illnesses such as acute nephritis, meningitis, or rheumatic fever, all of which can be fatal.

Sandra was given one dose of Chamomilla. Her mother took her home and she went to sleep early that evening. She slept through the night and woke up in a good mood, eating and drinking normally, back to her old self. She never needed another dose and soon her tonsils returned to normal.

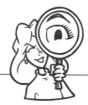

Curious Clues

You may be familiar with chamomile as a tea used for relaxation especially before bed. In large amounts, however, it can cause agitation and irritability. Patients who may benefit from homeopathic chamomile (Chamomilla) are well known for their incredible irritability and complaining. In addition, they have symptoms of ...

➤ Inflammation of tonsils with great swelling.

➤ Suppuration of tonsils (pus).

➤ Capricious, complaining.

➤ Shrieking with the pain.

➤ Desire to be carried.

➤ Dictatorial (bossy).

➤ Heedless, careless.

➤ Conscientious about trifles (likes things in order).

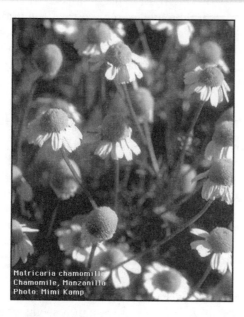

Matricaria chamomilla
Chamomile, Manzanilla
Photo: Mimi Kamp

Homeopathic Chamomilla is helpful for someone who is incredibly irritable, bossy, and wants to be held while complaining of her sore throat or tonsillitis.

183

Cough: The Hack Is Back

A cough is used by the body to blow out the air pipes of any foreign material or accumulated mucus. The protective reflex of coughing kicks in when the membranes lining the respiratory tract secrete excessive mucus or phlegm. These secretions help to protect your lungs from infection by trapping and flushing out viruses, bacteria, and other unwelcomed guests. The characteristic sudden burst of air helps to open the breathing passages and prevents infected mucus from falling back into your lungs.

A cough is not an illness but is a protective reflex. You will want to treat the underlying causes of the cough. With an infant, make sure you're not dealing with pertussis or whooping cough, which can be a serious illness for children. The adult population is about 90 percent susceptible to pertussis, which leads to chronic bronchitis. This can be easily passed on to children and others by coughing on them. A productive cough that expels sputum is rarely advised to be stopped or suppressed by cough medicines. The cough is doing its job. Conventional medicine uses a wide array of products that can be categorized into antitussives (stop cough) or expectorants (start cough). Homeopathic remedies seek to treat the underlying condition of a cough while bolstering your overall health and well-being. Good diagnostics should not be skipped, however, and seeking a qualified homeopath can help quiet your chronic cough.

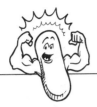

Potent Pellets

Answering these clues to your cough can let you or your health-care provider understand the possible cause:

➤ How often and how long do you cough?

➤ What type of material is being coughed up (mucus or blood)?

➤ What color is your sputum (white, clear, green, yellow)?

➤ What is the consistency of the material coughed up (thick, thin, frothy)?

➤ Does it hurt when you cough?

➤ What is the sound of your cough (rattle, barking, low pitched)?

Chronic Pediatric Cough (Presented by Savitri Clarke)

Lyle is an adorable five-year-old boy who sits on his mom's lap and hides his head on her chest. It is October and he is coming for help with a chronic cough. His mother begins: "Lyle gets croup every fall, winter and spring. It starts when the forced hot air heat gets turned on in the fall. It gets so bad that we must use steroids to open up his breathing passages. Once he had to go to the emergency room for a shot. He will say 'I can't breathe.' He seems to do well with it. We are the ones who get scared. He is stoic. He wants to tell mom he is sick but doesn't get panicked. The cough is dry and barky. After the first croup, Lyle started getting ear infections. Our only clue was he slowed down on his eating."

When I asked more about the cough Lyle's mom offered: "The cough wakes him up and he can't stop coughing. He gags but doesn't vomit though it seems like he is going to."

I asked Lyle what he likes to do. "I like to play with my super magnet. I test for everything that is metal. I would like to be a monster truck driver." "Why?" I asked. "Because you can jump all the jumps and it would be fun."

His mom says Lyle is very much a risk taker, fearless, loves the excitement. He doesn't think a lot. Just has fun in the moment. He is a daydreamer, goes with the flow. "Lyle loves to wrestle, fight, and be physical. He is very mechanical and likes to take things apart and put them back together. He doesn't care about being the center of attention. His feelings get hurt easily and he cries, such as if a boy doesn't always want to play with him. He has an intense reaction to feeling left out or rejected."

Lyle is very hot-blooded and doesn't like the sun. He loves Popsicles and will ask to suck on ice if he is hot from running around. He often says he has a tummy ache. He has a lazy streak and doesn't mind being dirty. He will lie on the floor and talk to himself, daydreaming. When you talk to him he blocks you out. He is a high-spirited boy who feels everything intensely, emotionally. He gets devastated easily and gets right back up again just as easily. He cares deeply about the family but could come down in the morning and be the only one who does not give me a hug, but he seems to need it the most. If his teacher reprimands him at school, it devastates him. He can become very detached and aloof, especially when he is sick." I gave him Natrum Sulphuricum.

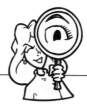

Curious Clues

At first glance, Lyle looked like a homeopathic Sulphur child. A hot-blooded, active, playful, high-spirited, mechanically oriented child with a lazy streak and a tendency to daydream. But the sensitivity to reprimand and rejection, his stoic reaction to pain, his detached aloofness, and his fearless risk-taking behavior coupled with his desire for ice made me decide on the remedy Natrum Sulphuricum. Adding the "Natrum" part makes it a salt, sodium sulphate, or Glauber's Salt. This remedy type includes many of the Sulphur characteristics, but adds the sensitivity of the "Natrum" to rejection and criticism with the tendency to be more closed about his feelings.

When Lyle came in for the follow-up one month later, he sat in his own chair and spoke right up. "I didn't get my throat clogged up like I did and I stopped coughing. My ears have been okay. Most of the things have changed. I used to get waist aches and I am not having them now." His mom agreed: "Those symptoms left almost immediately. I noticed a difference on the way home in the car. His eyes seemed more open right away. We have seen much more open communication at home. That was immediate. His sensitivity to reprimand is far lessened. All of this was immediate. Amazing!"

Lyle and his mom would have been happy just to see his chronic cough go away. But as a bonus, the child became more emotionally open and available. Homeopathy, such a gift!

Sinusitis: Pain in the Pockets

We've all got four pairs of sinus cavities or open spaces tucked away behind our cheeks, nose, and eyes. These sinus cavities produce mucus that carries away foreign particles, warms the air we breathe, and makes our heads a little lighter to lift. Unfortunately, between 30 million and 50 million Americans each year develop an infection in these air-filled pockets known as sinusitis (*-itis* at the end of any word means "inflammation"). Researchers believe as many as 14 percent of the country's population suffers from chronic sinusitis.

Colds, viruses, and allergies often leave your sinuses vulnerable to infection. Anatomical problems such as a deviated septum (a shift in the nasal cavity) or nasal polyps (small growths in the lining of the nose canals) block off sinus passages. Sinusitis may also result from an infected tooth, swimming, a disease or injury to the sinuses.

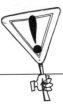

Caution Keeper

Normal colds or flus are caused by viruses that infect the nose and throat. Symptoms of nasal congestion, runny nose, post-nasal drip, cough, overall achiness, and fatigue separate these conditions from sinusitis. Colds typically last 7 to 10 days with no treatment necessary. If your sinuses still hurt and you're plugged up when the rest of you feels okay, you may have moved from a cold to sinusitis. Check with your health-care provider to be sure.

Sinusitis Symptoms

When sinuses get blocked and filled with fluid, bacteria can grow there and cause infection. The following symptoms can tip you off that you may have more than a cold:

➤ Feeling of fullness in the face

➤ Pressure behind the eyes

➤ Nasal obstruction, difficulty in breathing through your nose

➤ Postnasal drip

➤ A cold that won't go away

➤ Foul smell in your nose

➤ Loss of smell

➤ Fever

➤ Toothache

➤ Thick, yellow, foul-smelling nasal discharge

➤ Headache in the face or forehead

Antibiotics in conventional medicine are commonly prescribed to eliminate any bacteria that may be causing an infection. The challenge is to open the sinus passageways so that they can drain, while stimulating the immune system so that your body can resist future infections. Homeopathic medicines aim toward that goal without any side effects or weakening of your good bacteria. The next patient's story will help you understand how this mini—yet mighty—medicine can help you open and clear your sinuses.

Chronic Sinusitis (Presented by Savitri Clarke)

Joan is a 30-year-old woman who looks tired. She has dark circles under her eyes and flops down in my chair to talk. She begins, "I have a lot of allergies—to foods, especially wheat, and ragweed. My sinuses blow up and I get cranky, irritable. I get sinus infections easily. I tend to be low energy since I've had kids and my sex drive is also very low. I feel overwhelmed a lot with three kids."

Next Joan shares her history of anorexia in college when she was down to 90 pounds. While still on the slim side, she is 25 pounds heavier now. "I don't see food as nourishing but as fuel, I am a deprivation type. When it was really bad I used a lot of laxatives. I am addicted to sugar and have a hypoglycemic reaction to it. At first I get hyper then one hour later I become very irritable, a bear, impatient, bothered by noise. I need to eat every two hours."

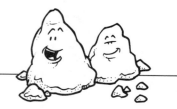

Natural Nuggets

There are many home treatments that can cut your sinus symptoms short:

➤ Take 30mg to 60mg of zinc a day.

➤ Take 15,000 IU of beta-carotene a day.

➤ Avoid mucus-producing foods such as dairy, sugars, and bananas.

➤ Avoid allergens such as tobacco smoke, dust, and auto fumes.

➤ Drink plenty of water, 8 to 10 eight-ounce glasses per day.

➤ Place alternating hot and cold wet washcloths on your face.

When I asked Joan about her emotional history she offered that her parents were very angry and her mother was emotionally withdrawn. "We were raised by a nanny. Mom left us crying a lot in our cribs. I could never do that with my kids. And my husband would like more sex. A lot of the time I just don't want to be touched."

She continues, "I am afraid of people's anger. I don't express my viewpoint until I test and make sure it is safe. When I am angry I want to throw things but I take a deep breath and talk to myself instead. I get irritable when my son cries. I don't know how to cry. I don't know what I am feeling a lot of the time."

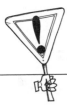

Caution Keeper

Antibiotics are commonly given during acute bouts of sinusitis, but are they really effective? According to a study reported by *The Lancet* (1997), antibiotic treatment did not improve the clinical course of acute maxillary sinusitis. They suggest alternative therapies could be another option.

With her sinus infections, her whole head swells up. It is very painful, especially if she has to stoop down to pick something up. It wears down her energy. She has dreams that she is underwater drowning. "I can see the surface but I can't get up there."

Joan's childhood was very repressive. Feelings were not respected or addressed at all. She didn't even know what she was feeling. She is sensitive to anger because of her parents' continued fighting. She was always afraid they would split up and someone would leave her. She has a history of mild colitis where she gets intestinal cramping and diarrhea. Joan was given the remedy Magnesium Muriaticum, homeopathic magnesium chloride.

Over the next several months, Joan's sinuses improved and she reported no sinus infections and only mild allergy symptoms. Her energy improved and her obsession with exercise moderated. Emotionally she felt more available to her children and her husband. She reports doing much better with feeding herself and feels she is "starting to have that mother inside of me to mother myself."

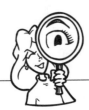

Curious Clues

People needing Magnesium Muriaticum lacked basic nurturing growing up. Their feelings are repressed and they feel very forsaken, alone, and untrusting of others who might hurt or disappoint them. As a result, they become independent, take care of themselves and others, but have trouble allowing others in at any deep level. They often have dreams about drowning which may represent their inability to deal with their emotions (represented by water). Anger is scary for this type because people might abandon them if they get angry. Sinuses and allergies are common as is any kind of cramping including menstrual cramping and intestinal cramping. This cramping is a physical manifestation of their cramped emotional state.

Asthma: A Hesitation of Respiration

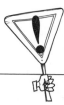

Asthma is becoming a major public health concern crisis in several Western nations, and the United States is no exception, where about 12 million people have asthma. The *Merck Manual* reports that from 1982 to 1992 the prevalence of asthma increased from 34.7 to 49.4 per 1,000 people. During the past 10 years, the death rate from asthma has increased 45 percent. In 1990 (the last recorded statistics), hospital care of asthmatics cost more than $2 billion while the total cost of asthma care was more than $6.21 billion. The rapid rise in asthma leads experts to believe the cost care dollars are now higher.

Asthma is a condition that blocks the flow of air into your lungs. During an asthma attack, spasms in the muscles surrounding the bronchi (small airways in the lungs) make the air passages smaller. This makes you feel like you have to fight for every breath by sucking air through these smaller openings. During an asthma attack, many people experience coughing, wheezing (the raspy sound as you breathe), shortness of breath, and a feeling of tightness in your chest.

Treatment for asthma in conventional medicine involves the use of drug therapy along with controlling environmental exposure to toxins. Education is a key factor in both conventional and homeopathic care. Ending the chronic cycle of suffering and limitations that asthma patients experience without the use of drugs that have numerous side effects is the goal in homeopathic treatment. I hope the patient's story that you are about to read will underscore the help that may await you working with a qualified homeopathic practitioner.

Chronic Asthma (Presented by Savitri Clarke)

Martha is a 45-year-old woman with a long history of asthma. She comes to see me while in the

Caution Keeper

Asthma spasms are commonly triggered by hypersensitivity to environmental factors. Typical triggers include …

➤ Animal dander.

➤ Tobacco smoke.

➤ Environmental pollutants.

➤ Weather changes.

➤ Extremes in dryness and humidity.

➤ Dust mites.

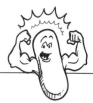

Potent Pellets

Urbanization, not race, is the main risk factor in asthma. A national data set of 17,110 children investigated the reasons for higher asthma among black children in the United States. Race did not heighten the risk, but both white and black children living in cities regardless of income were at significantly greater risk for asthma than nonurban children.

Source: American Journal of Critical Care Medicine, 2000

middle of getting a divorce. She describes her symptoms: "Frequent bronchitis, severe tightness in the chest so I can't breathe, and wheezing. I sneeze *a lot!* I have made many trips to the emergency room. I am very scared. For the last few years I have taken prednisone (a steroid) at the first sign of a cold. I know that isn't good for me long term. I am healthy but I have to work at it." She continues, "When I get sick I feel a chill between my breasts. I am always cold, especially my feet. Lately I have been losing my hair."

When I asked Martha more about her life she complained, "I resent that everything is a struggle for me. Other people seem to have it so much easier. I go to their houses and I can barely stand it. Why do they have such beautiful things?" Martha's divorce has not been easy. She expresses hatred of her husband and her resentment of her current financial situation. She lives in a wealthy suburb and money is always a struggle. She blames him for much of her unhappiness. "I have trouble with rage and fear. It is starting to get to me more. Friends are having to choose sides. It keeps bringing up more anger and resentment.

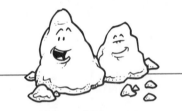

Natural Nuggets

Maintaining a healthy lifestyle can help reduce asthma symptoms. These include ...

➤ Omega fatty acids (fish like salmon or polyseed oil).

➤ Foods high in magnesium (apples, apricots, brown rice, avocados).

➤ Clean your air; change your furnace filters and try an air purifier.

➤ Wash sheets and blankets frequently in hot water to kill dust mites.

➤ Don't smoke or let anyone smoke around you.

"My mother was really a screwed-up person. I was convinced she didn't love me, but I didn't think she even liked me. I used to have a fantasy of getting adopted by somebody else. It was a bad match emotionally. My parents are not bad people, just that the stork delivered the wrong baby. I always felt if I had been delivered across the street it would have been fine."

About six months ago, Martha had an episode of very intense joint pain. "Just before the pain started I had gone to visit my friend Sara. Compared to my life her life is really easy. Not that I am begrudging her easy life, but I was struck with how much easier her life was. It was the first time I acknowledged that my life is hard. I don't like whining and I don't make a distinction between whining and acknowledging how hard it is. I live in a rich town. There are a lot of people to be jealous of."

I asked Martha how she thought others see her. "I am not warm. I am friendly, but there is this detached, emotionally aloof thing I do. I don't go around sharing my soul with a lot of people. If there is any thought of things getting emotional with a man I shut down. Besides, I have become so critical and cynical that I can't imagine ever living with anyone again."

She had a recurrent dream of being in a romantic kiss with her husband and realizing he had a gun to her temple. Then he pulls the trigger and she wakes up.

Martha was given Ammonium Muriaticum, or homeopathic ammonium chloride. In addition to fitting the above profile, Ammonium Muriaticum is associated with the following symptoms ...

➤ Chronic inflammation of the bronchial tubes.

➤ Respiration impeded with oppression in chest.

➤ Frequent sneezing.

➤ Coldness of the chest.

➤ Hair falling out, alopecia.

➤ Dreams of being shot.

➤ Envy.

➤ Hatred.

➤ Critical.

Martha called me one week later saying, "I am so surprised how much better I am already! My lungs feel clearer than they have in ages. And, though I didn't bring it up as a problem when we met, my sexual energy has returned! It's amazing!" Martha continued to improve with no incidence of respiratory problems for many months. She began to soften emotionally and became open to finding a new partner. She has noticed her feelings of resentment and envy have decreased dramatically, allowing her to finally find enjoyment in life.

Allergies: The Unpleasing Sneezing

Allergies are a major cause of illness in both children and adults. The National Institute of Allergy and Infectious Disease estimates between 40 million and 50 million Americans react to a multitude of substances from latex to peanuts to pollens. A *hay fever* attack, usually induced by wind-borne pollens, can extend the miserable symptoms of prolonged, often violent sneezing, itchy painful nose, throat, and roof of mouth, stuffy, runny nose and watery itchy eyes for as long as 15 to 20 minutes. These attacks can occur several times a day during the season your allergies are active.

Dose of Info

Allergic rhinitis, or **hay fever,** is characterized by allergic reactions to pollen, grasses, and other substances. These are two types: seasonal, which occurs only during the time of year when certain plants pollinate—February to fall; and perennial, which occurs all year-round.

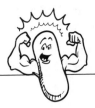

Potent Pellets

A news story has found that homeopathic dilutions may be as effective as topical steroids for treating allergies. A randomized, double-blind placebo-controlled study examined 50 patients with perennial allergic rhinitis. A 21 percent improvement in nasal airflow was noted in the homeopathic group with only 2 percent measured in the placebo group.

Source: British Medical Journal, 2000

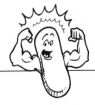

Potent Pellets

A nine-year-long study shows homeopathic treatment to be comparable with those of conventional antihistamines, but without any side effects. The authors of the report conducted 11 studies between 1980 and 1989 for patients suffering from acute allergies.

Source: Forsh Komplementärmed, 1996

At first it may seem that you have a cold; however, allergies do not come with a fever, and the usual discharge is runny and clear, instead of the yellow or green mucus that's typical of colds.

Conventional medical treatment of allergies combines avoidance of allergens with drug therapy. Many of these medications can cause drowsiness, and less often nausea, epigastric distress, and diarrhea. You must be alert to the possibility of drug interactions with other prescriptions you may be taking, and some drugs like ethanolamines are poorly tolerated by the elderly.

Homeopathic help for allergies offers treatment with no side effects, with the goal being to help strengthen your immune system, so that your body becomes less reactive to the allergic material that once bothered you. You'll see how this works in the next homeopathic story of the case of the cats.

Perennial Allergies: The King of Cats

Jim was a successful real estate broker with a potential problem. He was highly allergic to cats, any kind of short-hair, long-hair, tall, thin, or fat cat. Any cat—whether it was nestling around his legs or in another room—would create an allergic reaction with violent sneezing, runny nose, and sudden onset of watery, itchy, red eyes. This was driving him crazy. "I can tell if a cat is living or has ever lived in a home by my reactions. I'm trying to instill confidence in my clients, when I have to suddenly excuse myself. I don't know what to do!"

Jim told me about going through homes in and out of the snow and rainy weather, air-conditioning, and feeling like his body was being worn down by the parade of properties.

Jim had known success, but had lost it all over business. Losing a marriage and the custody of his daughter had deeply hurt him. He now concerned himself with his second marriage and new baby. "You come to know what is really valuable when you lose everything." He had definite opinions about how things should be done the second time around.

Chilliness and dampness seemed to provoke an old backache, stomach upset, and urgency in urination. I gave Jim the homeopathic formula Dulcamara.

The first follow-up had Jim very excited about homeopathic care. His allergic reactions had decreased significantly. It took him longer to begin to have symptoms, and they were less severe. I boosted the potency on his remedy and had him take it less often. The following month he noticed very few cat allergies, despite being around quite a few cats that month. He was feeling more secure about his family, relaxing around the whole idea of a loving life at home. A year follow-up proved that he had become a friend to all cats. They no longer bothered him. He could be around cats for extended periods of time and even began to pet and hold them. He was quite pleased and has not needed to repeat his remedy to keep his feline friends.

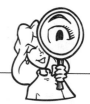

Curious Clues

Solanum Dulcamara is the diluted and succussed plant of the bittersweet nightshade. Jim's allergic symptoms combined with his very strong guardianship of his new family initially made me think of this remedy. This general aggravation from the cold and dampness, combined with the urgent urination and backache, gave me confidence this remedy would help him conquer his allergies with cats.

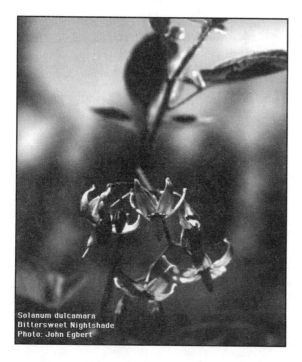

Solanum dulcamara
Bittersweet Nightshade
Photo: John Egbert

Dulcamara, the homeopathic form of the bittersweet nightshade, is useful for people suffering from allergies who are chilled easily, react poorly to dampness, and are preoccupied with family matters.

Being able to take a deep, clear breath is essential to our peace of mind. This chapter has shown you the homeopathic options for prolonging better breathing without the continued use of medications. Many families are opting to add homeopathics into a comprehensive wellness plan. Seek out a qualified homeopath to consult with about the help you are looking for.

The Least You Need to Know

➤ The homeopathic Chamomilla can be useful for treating tonsillitis in children who are bossy, irritable, careless, and have a desire to be carried.

➤ Covering your mouth when you cough is a simple way to prevent the spread of infected water droplets from being sprayed onto your family and friends.

➤ Homeopathic medicines are a safe, nontoxic way to help the 30 million to 50 million Americans who suffer from sinusitis.

➤ Urbanization, not race, is the main risk factor for developing asthma.

➤ During a nine-year study, homeopathic treatment of acute allergies was shown to be as effective as conventional antihistamines without the side effects.

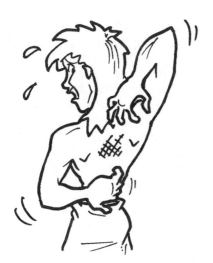

Chapter 17

Service for the Epidermis

In This Chapter

➤ Learn homeopathic solutions for acne

➤ Erase eczema with diluted solutions

➤ Discover homeopathic ways of treating stubborn psoriasis

➤ Get warts off with homeopathic medicines

➤ Treat poison ivy effectively and safely

Yes, homeopathic medicines have the potential to help you clear your skin. Right away? That all depends on the source of your vital force. Your skin is the largest organ you've got. It shrink-wraps your muscles, organs, and bones in a breathing, waterproof protective covering that stands up to sun, sand, and even tattoos! The skin will reflect the symptoms of your body, so it only makes sense to me that topical creams and ointments may at best suppress the symptoms temporarily, but offer no lasting effects. In great contrast, I've had many satisfied patients who've consulted me for chronic skin problems. It does take time, persistence, and patience, but the boost of health and lasting glow will be worth it.

Acne: A Barricade of Blemishes

It's a zit! What about senior pictures on Friday? This request for help from the heavens has been echoing around high schools for a long time. Acne is an inflammatory skin disorder that affects about 85 percent of Americans, to some degree, between the ages of 12 and 25. Acne is a natural consequence of growing up, for it is the higher levels of testosterone (male sex hormone that girls have, too!) that cause a gland at the bottom of every hair follicle to produce keratin and sebum. With the hormones raging, the overproduction of these oily substances lubricate all your hairs, even the tiny ones on your face, and usually clog up the follicles and the skin's pores. Bacteria multiply in the follicle, and the skin becomes inflamed. Sebaceous glands that do all the oiling are found in great numbers on the face, back, chest and shoulders, coincidentally the sites of most acne formation. These glands keep pumping out the oil like a Texas gusher, making your pores sticky and trapping bacteria. If the follicle is trapped near the surface, it's a white head; deeper clogs produce blackheads. Severe acne can result in lifelong scarring.

Treatment options in conventional medicine include an array of prescription and over-the-counter products. With an estimated 50 million Americans looking for solutions to their acne, products like face-cleaning systems, prescription benzoylperoxide facial wipes, antibiotic wipes, Retin-A cream, Accutane, and oral contraceptives lead the pack in possibilities. Homeopathic solutions can be an important part of a nontoxic plan to help your body eliminate waste without worry.

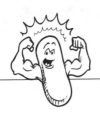

Potent Pellets

One of the functions of the skin is to eliminate a portion of your body's toxic waste products through sweating. Some doctors call the skin your "third kidney," because it helps the liver and kidney discharge toxins. As these toxins escape through the skin, they disrupt the skin's healthy integrity.

Source: Prescription for Nutritional Healing

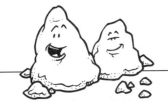

Natural Nuggets

Avoid stress for better skin. Stress can increase hormone output and cause acne flare-ups. Try getting at least 15 minutes a day of sunshine, along with regular exercise and sufficient sleep.

Acne: Healing Skin from Within (Presented by Savitri Clarke)

When Frank enters my office he seems curious but insecure about what is to come. He is a 45-year-old man who developed typical acne at age 14, the onset of puberty. As he got older he would get rashes on his face when he would exercise or eat certain foods. A year ago he had a severe outbreak. "My face was all inflamed, broken out, eyes and cheeks were swollen to the point that it started to block my vision a little. I was under a lot of work stress at the time. It was a terrible time for me. I took antibiotics and that cleared it up." During this outbreak he was diagnosed with acne rosacea. Since then Frank's skin has gone through recurrent cycles of severe outbreaks. Cortisone cream used to help but now has little effect. He had used it for 20 years to take care of little rashes on his face that were diagnosed as eczema and seborrhea. The antibiotics were clearly not working either so he decided to try homeopathy.

When I asked Frank to describe his nature, he says, "I am very much a moral person, a very straight person. You know how kids can be really horrible when someone looks funny or acts funny. I never joined in on that. I've always been sensitive to that." I asked Frank if that had ever happened to him. He remembers, "I had a problem with my speech when I was young. I couldn't pronounce a lot of words so I didn't want to raise my hand. I always worried about being picked by the teacher to say something. The kids would laugh if I had to read a paragraph. I hated that. I am more of a private person and now this skin condition has made me more that way."

"My father was very critical. I don't get along with him. He does things that makes you very mad, puts people down. He says things to people that make you want to crawl under the table. It embarrasses me. It has really hurt my confidence. I never cry. My wife says I should go with my gut when making decisions but I don't trust it. I think too much." I gave him Baryta Sulphuricum.

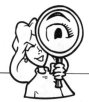

Curious Clues

Frank is a warm-blooded person but enjoys the heat. His skin gets worse when he is overheated, especially when he is hot enough to perspire. Frank seemed like a typical Sulfur type:

➤ Warm-blooded, skin worse from getting overheated

➤ Intellectualizes, suppresses emotions

➤ Easily embarrassed, with flushing of face

➤ History of many skin eruptions, often suppressed with medications

➤ Much theorizing, overthinking

➤ Lack of self-confidence

In addition to the above, Frank had a history of and sensitivity to being mocked, laughed at, and put down. This, coupled with his overall sense of insecurity, led me to give him Baryta Sulphuricum, or homeopathic barium sulphate.

After a dose of Baryta Sulphuricum, Frank's skin got worse for a week and then started to heal. He was able to eat the foods that previously aggravated his skin. Over the next year his skin improved by at least 90 percent and continues to do so. As his fear of being laughed at and put down decreased, he began to feel more secure and confident at work and out in the world.

Eczema: The Bake and Flake Skin

Eczema is also known as atopic dermatitis and affects between 3 percent and 7 percent of our population. In more than 70 percent of patients, it runs in the family. The skin typically becomes dry, flaking, scaling, and thickening. It also often changes color, and itching can develop.

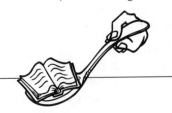

Dose of Info

According to *A Dictionary of Word Origins*, the word **eczema** originated with the Greek metaphoric word *ekzema* meaning *eruption* or *boiling over*. Other descriptive Indo-European bases include the Sanskrit word *yas* (*boil, foam*), Welsh *ias* (*boiling*), and English *yeast*.

Eczema occurs most often on the face, wrists, elbows, and knees, but it is not limited to those areas. You're likely to discover it on your newborn baby or infant, although many of those children outgrow it before their second birthdays. If they do not, they are likely to be chronic sufferers with distinctive thickened brownish-gray skin where the outbreaks frequently occur.

Conventional care uses corticosteroid creams or ointments applied three times daily. Because these products can be expensive, white petrolatum, hydrogenated vegetable oil, hydrophilic petroleum (avoid if allergic to lanolin) are recommended. Adrenal suppression may be experienced if high potency corticosteroid creams are used for prolonged, widespread use. Homeopathic treatment focuses on the patterns that are systemically coating the dry scaly skin.

Chronic Eczema (Presented by Savitri Clarke)

Tara is a cheerful 39-year-old woman who comes seeking help for severe eczema on her hands. As we enter the consultation room she trips a little on the carpet and immediately apologizes. As we sit down I clumsily drop some papers on the floor and she again apologizes. She seems polite to a fault. She shows me her hands, which are extremely inflamed, cracked, and raw. She says, "They itch to the point where I can't stand it. They get vesicles that break open. When it is bad, it is crippling—I can't move my hands. It is cyclical, worse before my period. I am allergic to Quaternium 14, which is in hair products and cosmetics, also hair dye, nickel, and formaldehyde. It started on my palms and has moved to my fingers now. I also get cold sores on my lips."

Tara is a dental hygienist and works in gloves. She is angry because she has been told she must change her profession. Her eczema started three years ago when her husband was out of work. She had a one-year-old child, and was forced to work full-time and rely on others to take care of her daughter while her husband looked for a job.

The year before the eczema started Tara was very angry that her husband lost his job "but I felt fortunate that I could go back to work and support the family. I tried to focus on the bright side—that is who I am. I helped my husband feel safe so he could do what he needed to do."

198

Emotionally her skin problem didn't affect Tara until the last six months. "I kept getting false hopes that my skin would clear. What is it I am not doing?" Tara starts to tear up but chokes it back. She is obviously feeling upset and desperate but is uncomfortable showing that to me.

Before her period, Tara's skin gets worse: "I get sad and weepy then. I know at that time of the month I shouldn't make decisions."

Tara is a very empathetic person. "I help others at my own risk. If they are receptive that is fine. The minute I feel they aren't, I pull back. Why waste the energy? I tend to take on more than is mine. I do for others, I am a helper. I feel good when I can help others."

Recently Tara was involved with a very upsetting situation at work when she was blamed for things she hadn't done. "I knew in my heart I hadn't done those things. I really felt betrayed." Her skin got much worse after that.

I chose for her the remedy Natrum Carbonicum, which is homeopathic sodium carbonate. People who benefit from this remedy are independent, very responsible, helpful, caring, and reserved with their emotions. They often have deep emotional injuries from having been betrayed. They feel hurt easily and tend to shut down. They are almost always cheerful, tending to not show their negative feelings. They have trouble asking for help and do not want to burden others with their problems.

They bear their grief silently. Tara fits this description well. Her skin problems began after her husband's company betrayed them (after all they had done for the company) and then was reaggravated with the betrayal at work (after all she had done for her boss).

Tara's hands cleared nicely for more than a month. Then she had an upset at work and had a minor flare-up. Soon after that she returned for her six-week follow-up and we repeated her remedy. Her skin has continued to improve.

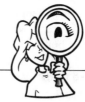

Curious Clues

The remedy Natrum Carbonicum is associated with symptoms of ...

➤ Vesicular eruptions on fingers with cracking and itching.

➤ Vesicular eruptions on the lips.

➤ Itching worse from getting hot.

➤ Sad and weepy before the period.

Psoriasis: Developing Thick Skin

Psoriasis varies in severity from one or two patches of silvery scaly skin to widespread dermatosis with red areas on the legs, knees, elbows, scalp, ears, and back. In about 30 percent to 50 percent of people, fingernails and toenails can be discolored and develop ridges and pits, looking similar to a fungal infection. The cause is unknown,

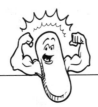

Potent Pellets

The underlying cause of psoriasis is unknown, but there are current theories. Since psoriasis is rare in countries where the diet is low in fat, a faulty use of fat may be involved. Current research also points to an immune system role since people with HIV or AIDS often have severe psoriasis. The buildup of toxins in an unhealthy colon has also been linked to the development of psoriasis.

Source: Prescription for Nutritional Healing

but the thick scaling has traditionally been attributed to increased epidermal growths that never mature. Psoriasis is often hereditary, and begins over a wide range of 10 to 40 years of age, but no age is exempt.

Treatment with conventional medicine first involves the use of the simple agents such as lubricants, topical corticosteroids, and topical vitamin D derivatives. Exposure to sunlight is usually beneficial. Once these have failed or the condition is more severe or systemic, powerful antimetobolite such as methotrexate and immunosuppressive drugs are employed. A new study conducted by researchers at Wake Forest University School of Medicine reported that due to the side effects with pregnant women using oral medications, men are three times more likely to receive powerful drugs for severe psoriasis. Systemic corticosteroid should also be avoided due to their side effects.

Homeopaths seek to end the cycle of psoriatic flare-ups with treatments that focus on healing your entire system. Psoriasis is not an easy condition to treat, but the rewards of a successful nontoxic homeopathic treatment can be a lasting solution for those that suffer from this sickening thickening of the skin.

Psoriasis: The Amazing Scratching Man

"Once I start scratching a spot, it will spread to the whole limb," said 27-year-old Jason when he visited my office for a consultation for his psoriasis. He leaned toward me describing with great detail the patches of dark scaly skin on his fingers, buttocks, back, wrists, behind his knees, arms, elbows, and inside his thighs. Itching would wake him up at night where he usually found he had scratched the lesions until they bled. He had been given a range of medication and topical lotions, had changed detergents and soaps, but nothing had helped. He currently uses special sensitive skin soaps and applies baby oil after a shower.

"I'm up-to-date on the world, financially and politically. I'm in tune with what people want. I have a huge promotional plan that I need to get going. I'm maxed out on my credit cards, but I will eventually be rewarded."

When Jason was 20, his father tried to get him into an apprenticeship with a union job. "I had to get out, I'm more of a stage performer. I live more consciously than 80 percent of the people on earth." At this point, I'm trying to understand Jason who sits in front of me in a jean jacket outfit with his shirt collars turned up (with heavily oiled hair like in a 1950s biker's movie). "I'm hot all the time, but I control it. I take charge of my own environment. I'm not in a relationship now, because I don't know any balanced women. I have to be careful who influences me. I'm one of the most balanced people I've ever met. I'm going to be America's next superhero. I'm going no place but up!" I gave Jason the homeopathic remedy Sulphur.

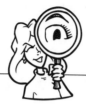

Curious Clues

Jason exhibited many of this famous polycrests (many uses) keynotes in a rather strong way. He kept telling me how incredible he was (rubric: bragging), how smart and intellectual he had become during his life (rubrics: egotism, philosophical, theorizing). Other Sulphur symptoms are ...

➤ Psoriasis.

➤ Eruptions, itchy worse at night.

➤ Relationships and sex can be seen as a distraction.

➤ Warm-blooded, worse from heat.

➤ Egotism and bragging.

➤ Laziness, talks a lot, but accomplishes little in reality.

➤ Intellectual, theorizing.

➤ Extroverted, bossy, in charge.

➤ Antibiotics.

➤ Critical of others.

Almost immediately, Jason was helped by this remedy. His skin lesions lessened over the next few months (as did the superman personality). He became truly more balanced and went on to do stable businesses and live comfortably.

I heard from Jason five years later when he brought his fiancée in for a consultation. He had not had a psoriasis flare-up for more than four years and was very content with his life.

Warts: I've Got You Under My Skin

Warts are small growths on the skin that are caused by at least 60 types of human papillomaviruses (HPV). After acne, they are the most common dermatological complaint with an estimated three out of four people developing a wart at some time in their lives. Warts can appear at any age, but are most frequent in older children and uncommon in the elderly. They can appear singly or in clusters, with most warts found on the hands, fingers, elbows, forearms, knees, face, and the skin around nails.

Plantar Warts (Presented by Savitri Clarke)

Julia is a nine-year-old little girl who appeared coy and cute with a clear desire to be liked. She has over 50 plantar warts covering the bottom of her feet, which hurt when she walks as if there is something sticking into her foot. She has had this pain for six months. She also has seasonal allergies this spring for the first time.

When asked to describe her nature, Julia says "I get nervous before school, because I am afraid I forgot my homework. I am scared if my father takes out the garbage and doesn't tell me."

Her father offers: "Julia can be whiny and clingy. She can be cautious physically and is not a risk taker. She still hides behind us in new situations! She writes a lot of stories about witches, morbid and violent stories. She also writes about mean kids that mistreat other kids. She seems particularly sensitive to that. She is very funny and likes to be funny. She does funny things with her eyebrows and makes her eyeballs go around. She has a strong sense of morality. Her friends tease her a lot. She is reserved but she uses it as a flirtation device that brings people to her. She doesn't like showoffs and will tell me not to act silly in public because it embarrasses her. She can get 'little' with her speech when away from us as if she will be cuter that way, trying hard to be liked."

Her mother adds, "Julia is not as confident as she would like to be. She has a lot of self-doubt and is very self-critical when she can't do something. She doesn't like sleeping over at her friends' houses but is afraid if she doesn't, she won't look grown up like the other girls."

When I asked about her physical development, an extraordinary symptom was revealed. Julia was physically tentative and walked late at 19 months. She literally walked on her knees for a long time as if she were aware she could fall easily and wasn't going to do it.

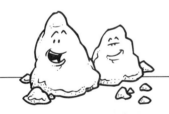

Natural Nuggets

My grandmother's folk remedy for warts: On the night of a full moon, rub an old penny on your warts. Place the penny in the center of a potato and bury it in your backyard when the moon is full and bright. By the next morning, your warts should be gone. So the story goes!

The parents then explain how Julia cries if there is a blowup between them. If there is tension between the parents, Julia will say, "What is going on here with you two? Please don't fight, do it for me because I don't want to live with this kind of tension." The mother said, "It is as if it threatens the security of our home and she can't evaluate the seriousness of it." Julia was given Baryta Carbonica, or homeopathic barium carbonate.

Baryta Carbonica fit well, as Julia feels insecure and clings to her parents for fear that she could lose their support. She is afraid of new people and things and is sensitive to being laughed at or mocked. When under stress she becomes more childish, even talking baby talk. She also has a strong aversion to bananas and an aversion to bathing, which are included in this remedy type.

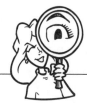

Curious Clues

Besides being a great remedy for painful plantar warts, Baryta Carbonica also has the following symptoms:

➤ Delusion that she walks on her knees (which she actually did!)

➤ Feeling laughed at, mocked

➤ Hiding

➤ Fear of strangers

➤ Jesting

➤ Embarrassed easily

➤ Childishness

One month later, Julia arrived with her parents for her follow-up visit. Both her plantar warts and her allergies disappeared after the remedy. Over the next two years, Julia received three doses of her remedy. She is growing up, is less dependent and clingy, less cautious, and less sensitive to embarrassment. Her parents, who had wondered if this child would ever grow up, are thrilled that she is emotionally stronger, more secure, and less fearful.

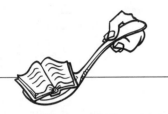

Dose of Info

Sensitivity to poison ivy or the irritating substance **urushiol** found in the oily sap is acquired. Your immune system is the most sensitive during childhood, but an estimated 65 percent of Americans remain sensitive to the plant. Light sensitivity is an indication that you may also be susceptible to poison ivy.

Poison Ivy: Scratching My Way Back to You, Babe

I hear stories of poison ivy that usually begin with, "We wanted to finally clear out the back part of our yard," or, "The kids were playing in the woods," and what follows is the story of a burning, itching rash with swelling, oozing, crusty blisters. About two million people a year join you in the seemingly endless itching.

Urushiol, the irritating substance in the poison ivy's leaf's stem, is one of the most potent toxins around. Less than an ounce is usually all that's needed to cause the familiar blisters, swelling, and itchiness. The plant is toxic even after it is dead or dried out.

Touching the plant, particularly in the spring or early summer when it's full of toxic sap, is the most common way to get in trouble. The poison sap can also be spread to your face, limbs, or genitals by touching them while the sap is still on your hands. Scratching can also spread the inflammation to other parts of your body. Petting an animal or using gardening tools that have the contaminated sap on them is another common way to pick up poison ivy.

Learning to recognize this poisonous plant can prevent an unpleasant scratching session. The old camp saying "leaflets three, let it be," is only partially true, because this family of poisonous plants grows in leaf patterns of three, five, seven, and nine. Learn what's most common in your area.

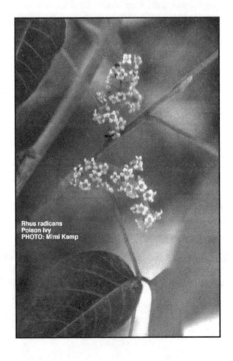

Rhus radicans
Poison Ivy
PHOTO: Mimi Kamp

The first action to take if you suspect you've been exposed is to carefully remove your clothes immediately, and wash the exposed skin with soap and water. Washing your skin within 5 to 10 minutes of exposure greatly reduces your chance of an allergic reaction. Make sure you also wash off your clothing, tools, gloves, and shoes. The oil can be toxic to you for about three weeks.

Mild reactions are treated by conventional medicine using topical hydrocortisone creams or oral antihistamines to help relieve itching. If symptoms are more severe, topical or oral steroids may be used to help with symptoms. Homeopathic treatment focuses on relieving itching and inflammation, while seeking to reduce or eliminate allergic sensitivities to poison ivy.

Next, take a look at the story of the little girl who used homeopathy to feel better inside and out.

Pediatric Poison Ivy

A 4½-year-old named Emily came into my office with her mother looking for solutions for repeated poison ivy reactions. Last year, Emily endured five separate exposures despite her mom's best efforts. The summer had barely begun and Emily was on her second reaction. She had poison ivy eruptions on her ankles, legs, and the bottom of her feet. Her poor little legs were swollen, bumpy, red, and itchy. Emily's mother had her using topical creams and even steroids and wanted to look for another way. She had even tried using a homeopathic remedy she picked up at the store, but it had not helped. A friend I had treated for poison ivy recommended homeopathy.

Emily's mother described her as an intense, impulsive little girl. "She switches back and forth from Dr. Jekyll to Mr. Hyde." I noticed during the interview that Emily taunted her little sister, walked behind her, and punched her hard, then quickly skipped away while her sister screamed. Emily likes to play with older kids, and she can hold her own. "She wants to be in charge and will tell the older kids what to do," her mother states. "She has no physical boundaries. Sometimes she's so sweet, the next minute she's in your space creating havoc."

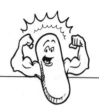

Potent Pellets

Poison ivy, oak, and sumac are commonly referred to as poison ivy. East of the Rocky Mountains, poison ivy is widespread, with poison oak common in the West and Southwest. Poison sumac is found in southern swamps and northern wetlands.

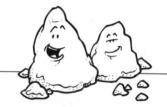

Natural Nuggets

The toxin in poison ivy, urushiol, does not affect dogs or cats, but they can get it on their fur and pass it on to you. If you suspect your pet has been running or rolling in poison ivy, wash it thoroughly (wear rubber gloves) and wash your own clothing afterward.

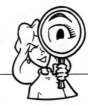

Curious Clues

Have you been keeping track of clues in Emily's case? What symptoms stick out as being common to poison ivy, and which ones are particular to this little girl? For Emily, I used these criteria to decide on Anacardium:

➤ Sensitivity to poison ivy or oak

➤ Two-sided personality; devil on one shoulder and an angel on the other

➤ Tendency toward being cruel and cold-hearted

➤ Inferiority that can come out as bossy or controlling due to the fear of letting others control them

➤ Internalized anger often from abuse or violence

➤ Desire to prove themselves with older kids

Emily's mother told me that Emily was surrounded by abuse, neglect, and violence in the first part of her life. She has a cruel side that can alternate with switching back to a little angel. She has outbursts of anger when she says bad words she's heard before. I gave Emily Anacardium Occidentale, the homeopathic remedy made from cashew.

Emily's mom called me to inform me that her daughter's poison ivy was gone in a couple of days. Her personality was still intense. We used Anacardium over the next year. This helped Emily to even out her emotions and move past her cruel edge. She also has not had a poison ivy reaction in more than two years despite being a healthy, active, adventurous little girl.

Homeopathy can be a great help for the inside or outside maladies that face us in daily life. These stories have illustrated how skin conditions can hold a physical and emotional charge, and be greatly alleviated by using solid homeopathic principles and accurate prescribing.

The Least You Need to Know

➤ Banish blemishes with homeopathic treatment.

➤ Stubborn eczema can be erased by using homeopathics like Natrum Carbonicum.

➤ Homeopathic medicine can help you put out the flare-ups of psoriasis.

➤ There are more than 60 different types of human papillomaviruses (HPV) that cause warts; you can remove them with nontoxic homeopathic treatments.

➤ Clear away poison ivy symptoms by using homeopathic medicines.

Part 4

Healing with Homeopathy

Although you may have been diagnosed with a common complaint, you'll find there's nothing "common" about the impact it has on your life. Homeopathy specializes in finding out the individual and unique qualities that you exhibit while you try to get well. This part of the book goes deeper into our discomfort with constricting constipation, heartburn, and other glitches of our gut. I'll also take you through homeopathic solutions for the persistent pains of headaches, bursitis, arthritis, and sciatica. Learn to loosen the limits on your lifestyle by using homeopathic medicines for such conditions as insomnia, high blood pressure, diabetes, mononucleosis, and fibromyalgia. We'll look at the role homeopathy plays in supporting your system when you're dealing with cancer. Read ahead to discover how your individuality is finally given voice in the medical system of homeopathy.

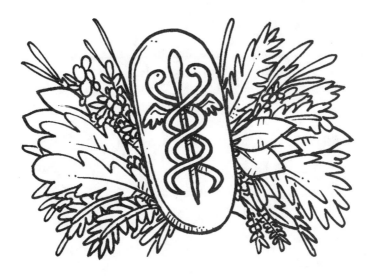

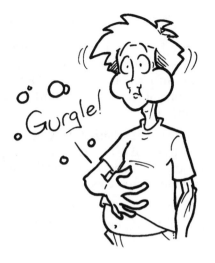

Chapter 18

Gastrointestinal Upsets

In This Chapter

➤ Put out the fire of heartburn with healing homeopathics

➤ Find homeopathic solutions to clear constipation

➤ Discover how to deal with diarrhea

➤ Learn about homeopathic help for irritable bowel syndrome

Your digestive tract is a bustling thoroughfare of specialized shops designed to process food along the stops. Every time we sit down for a meal, grab a quick sandwich, or snack on the run, we alert our busy broadway that guests have arrived to take the tour. Food and drink are transformed into a semi-liquid, gruel-like material called chyme. This can be absorbed by the body and used for fuel and energy. Most of us have had bouts of digestive distress which, as they say, "passes" quickly through the system.

In this chapter, I'm going to show you helpful homeopathic options for when your GI shop doors are closed. These are conditions that, while not life threatening, do have an enormous impact on the quality and comfort of your life. Since many of the symptoms are fairly common, pay close attention to the cases that reflect the unique features that make an accurate remedy selection possible. Keep in mind how homeopathy views you as a special and unique individual, capable of complete healing given the proper guidance. Enjoy your stroll through the nutritional neighborhood.

Heartburn: Reflux Deluxe

Do you enjoy your meals, but dread the next one or two hours of burning pain and pressure in your chest? You're probably suffering from *gastroesophageal reflux disease* (*GERD*), the term applied to what's often been called heartburn or acid reflux. More than 60 million American adults put up with this burning at least once a month, and about 25 million adults get a daily dose of fiery discomfort.

You may be one of the 25 percent of pregnant women who complain of daily heartburn, with more than 50 percent having occasional distress. GERD in infants and children is more common than originally recognized and researchers theorize that it may contribute to recurrent vomiting, coughing, respiratory problems, or failure to thrive.

There may be some concern with the burn because of mistaking heartburn for a heart attack. Exercise usually aggravates a heart attack and rest may relieve the pain. Heartburn pain is less likely to be affected by physical activity.

Dose of Info

In normal digestion, the lower esophageal sphincter (LES) opens to allow food to pass from the throat and esophagus (tube from the throat) into the stomach and closes to prevent food and acidic stomach juices from flowing back into the esophagus. **GERD** (or **gastroesophageal reflux disease**) occurs when the LES is weak or relaxes, allowing stomach stuff to flow back up into the esophagus. Feel the burn?

The Do's and Don'ts of Acid Reflux

There are several tips to follow while you try consulting a professional to relieve the reflux:

Do's

➤ Eat less and chew thoroughly at mealtime; when you swallow, food should already be slushy and liquefied.

➤ Eat your last meal two or three hours before bedtime; this will lessen the acid in your stomach when you lay down.

➤ Obesity contributes to this condition; losing weight often decreases symptoms.

➤ Stop smoking; cigarette smoking weakens the lower esophageal sphincter (LES), which needs to be strong to keep out stomach acids.

➤ Elevate the head of your bed about six inches or sleep on special wedges, which reduces heartburn by making stomach acid reflux more difficult due to gravity.

Don'ts

➤ Foods and beverages that weaken the LES include chocolate, peppermint, fried or fatty foods, coffee, or alcoholic beverages.

➤ Foods and beverages that can irritate the damaged lining of your esophagus include citrus fruits and juices, tomato products, and pepper.

Conventional treatment often includes antacids to neutralize stomach acids or H2 blockers, which inhibit acid secretion in the stomach. Long-term use of antacids can result in side effects such as diarrhea, change the way your body breaks down and uses calcium, or could have a buildup of magnesium, which is serious for patients who have kidney stones.

Homeopathy seeks to put out the fire in your gut for good. I'll share a patient's story that can show you the possibilities that homeopathic treatment may hold for you.

Heartburn (Presented by Savitri Clarke)

Deborah has been suffering for many years with heartburn. She is now taking Prilosec, which eliminates the symptom, but she doesn't like the chronic headaches that have replaced it. She comes looking for another way.

Deborah has fought weight her whole life. She had a history of bulimia for 12 years. "My mother was a great French cook, a stick of butter on everything. I loved it!" "I have always thought I was fat." The heartburn started 16 years ago when I was pregnant. I feel a burning, and I regurgitate food easily after I've eaten it." Wine and stimulants make the acid worse.

I asked Deborah about her emotions. "I was in a very abusive marriage. I reacted to him by having headaches, heartburn, and bulimia. I kept thinking he would change. My mother abused me emotionally, also. I served her, constantly gave to her, and even on her deathbed she couldn't say she loved me. My father was very quiet. He didn't know how to communicate. I hated listening to them argue. She would put him down. I always wanted to please him. We never talked about feelings." Deborah describes herself as a giver. "I could slip into being compulsive. I could gamble too much. I love to buy gifts."

In addition to regular heartburn, Deborah also has problems with pain in her left groin that would feel like she had dislocated her hip. She easily gets calf cramps and wakes at 3 A.M. since menopause even though she has started estrogen replacement therapy because of hot flashes. I gave her Magnesium Sulphuricum.

Deborah returned six weeks later. This is how she describes the changes: "I feel great. My heartburn is 90 percent better. I stopped the Prilosec and the headaches are almost gone. My leg cramps are much better, too!" Over the next year, Deborah became more confident, less needy, and began to feel deserving in a relationship. She is excited that she has finally found a wonderful partner and has plans to marry.

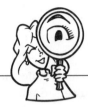

Curious Clues

At first, Deborah seemed like a typical Sulphur. She was warm-blooded with a flushed face and history of hot flashes, overly generous, and had heartburn. But Sulphur didn't cover the feelings of being unloved by her mother and the anxiety she felt whenever people were angry. Instead she was given Magnesium Sulphuricum or homeopathic magnesium sulphate. This remedy covers the unloved feeling, her strong need to please, and her willingness to accept the crumbs that both her mother and husband would give her. This remedy also covers the 3 A.M. waking, a dislocated feeling in the hip, and a tendency to get cramps in the muscles.

Constipation: A Plugged Pipeline

A walk down your local drugstore aisle or channel surfing will confirm that our society feels plugged up. Our bothersome bowels are not moving as often or as completely, giving us the condition of chronic *constipation*.

Dose of Info

According to *A Dictionary of Word Origins*, **constipation** is the original Latin word meaning "condition of being closely packed or compressed." At first the term was used literally as in "my, your garage looks constipated." Its English use as a medical term did not become popular until the mid-sixteenth century.

Lifestyle is often a likely candidate for concern in that lack of exercise, fluids, and fiber are often at the center of sluggish bowels. There is no correct number of bowel movements to have per week, although some experts feel a daily movement is important while others believe that regularity may depend on your individual history.

Eating high-fat meals, dairy, eggs, rich desserts, and sweets high in refined sugars is linked to causes of constipation. Some medicines such as antidepressants, antacids containing aluminum or calcium, antihistamines, diuretics, and anti-Parkinson's disease drugs can also lead to constipation.

Conventional medical therapies for constipation include laxatives, bulking agents to provide fiber to your colon, wetting agents to soften and bulk up stools, and enemas. Finding the cause of constipation is important; however, often it goes unexplained in conventional medical theories. Homeopathy recognizes that constipation is a symptom, not the illness, and seeks to use it as an important indicator when choosing accurate remedies. The next patient's story will show you how one family successfully used homeopathic treatment to dramatically improve the life of their son.

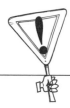

Caution Keeper

Misuse of laxatives and enemas can be harmful and habit forming. Your body begins to rely on the laxatives to bring on a bowel movement and forgets how to do its job by itself.

Pediatric Constipation

Jack was a two-year-old who had great difficulty with moving his bowels. His mother said he would stand, straighten out his legs, clench his fists, shake, and grit his teeth while straining to push a stool out. He would often scream as he passed painful bowel movements that were small hard balls of feces. Jack's mother said she had a great pregnancy, calm and happy, a normal natural birth, and their child had not received any vaccinations or fluoride drops. He was breast-fed for three months and had to go on formula because she could not supply enough milk. Jack had been constipated even on breast milk.

Throughout the two years before I first saw Jack, his parents had tried fruit juices, liquids, bran, and bottles of prune juice. They had to quit fruit juices, because of sudden advanced tooth decay. At age 1½, he had four fillings and several caps put on his teeth. He also developed an eczema-like rash on his face and hands. They also tried flaxseed, castor, and olive oils, along with butter and probiotic bacteria. None of these solutions were helpful long term.

When I asked both his parents about his personality, they said, "He likes order, not chaos. He needs routine and doesn't like change. He can be very focused, and likes to sit by himself and play. He doesn't play so much with other kids, or if he does, he lets them have their way. He's the one that is hit; he never kicks or hits others. He has a logical mind; he'd match shapes and colors. When he plays with his cars, he lines them all up in a row according to length and color."

I found his mother had a tendency toward constipation and most of Jack's organization skills she recognized as her own traits. I gave Jack Calcaria Silicate.

A six-week follow-up showed that his rash was gone, and Jack's parents reported he strained less. His stools were softer and easier to pass. He started to want to go places. On the next six-week visit, he passed normal stools, was happy, and more outgoing. Jack progressed normally over the next four years without an incident of constipation or eczema, became more interactive, and balanced in his behavior.

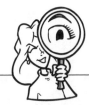

Curious Clues

Calcaria Silicate is used during the process of hardening concrete. This child's blockage was busted by recognizing some traits that are a unique match between the remedy and Jack. I rely on parents to give me emotional characteristics about their child. Their observations are key to learning the rest about the wee one's physical and emotional life. For Jack, these signs led me to check Calcaria Silicate:

➤ Passive, doing what other kids want

➤ Withdrawn, timid, fragile

➤ A homebody

➤ Many dental problems

➤ Constipation with hard stools, may even slip back

➤ Eczema

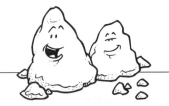

Natural Nuggets

The BRAT diet is recommended for treatment of diarrhea with children who have begun eating solid foods: **B**ananas; **R**ice; **A**pplesauce; **T**oast. Avoiding fats and sweets will also help to subside their rumbling insides.

Diarrhea: Panic for the Potty

Diarrhea describes bowel movements that are loose and watery. Sixty percent to ninety percent of stool weight is water and when it goes too high, you know it. Abdominal pain and cramping, sense of urgency to have a bowel movement, and sometimes nausea or vomiting are the clues you'll get if you have mild diarrhea.

Severe diarrhea may be a sign of serious illness with blood, mucus, or undigested food in your stool, weight loss or fever. Contact your health-care provider promptly if these severe symptoms persist longer than 24 hours. Losing all this fluid can deplete much-needed water and salts that your body needs to function. Keep drinking water to replace lost fluids.

Traveler's Diarrhea: More Than a Souvenir

According to a new report from the University of Zurich in Switzerland, about two out of three of us will develop traveler's diarrhea during two-week stays at high-risk destinations. Researchers say the old adage, "Don't drink the water," is still good advice, but their study suggests few tropical travelers follow this advice.

Results from the Swiss study found that 61 percent returning from India, 66 percent from Kenya, 38 percent from Jamaica, and 20 percent who traveled to Brazil returned with traveler's diarrhea. Researchers suggest that food safety rules be followed at all times when traveling. After all, you paid for the view of the beach, not the bathroom!

Diarrhea is a symptom, so whenever possible, it is best to learn the underlying cause of the commotion. Conventional medicine treats the colon with drugs to slow down the bowel such as diphenoxylate, codeine phosphate, or anticholinergics. Fluid replacement is also a standard procedure. Homeopathic treatment can be extremely effective in both acute situations and chronic cases, as you will see from the next patient's story.

Chronic Diarrhea (Presented by Savitri Clarke)

Joanne comes requesting treatment for intestinal problems. She describes herself as a "hysterical female pushing 50." She continues, "I don't know what's wrong with me. My intestines are very sensitive. Things I eat give me diarrhea. I had an operation when I was 40 for ulcerative colitis. They took out a huge part of my intestinal tract. I would eat something and have instant diarrhea; it ripped up my intestines. Since then I fall into bouts of it." In addition, Joanne gets sporadic migraines that seem to be hormonal and blood sugar–related. If she overworks and doesn't eat, she gets a headache. She goes on to talk about her irregular

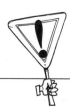

Caution Keeper

High-risk travel foods include tap water, ice cubes, dairy products, rare meat, seafood, and salads. Follow the rule of "boil it, cook it, peel it, or forget it" to avoid bringing back more than you bargained for from your travels!

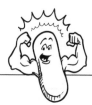

Potent Pellets

Five million children worldwide die every year from acute diarrhea. A Nepal study suggests that using homeopathic remedies alongside conventional oral rehydration therapy (ORT) can help acute diarrhea in young children. ORT only helps dehydration, while the combination treatment improved 85 percent of the cases.

Source: The Journal of Alternative and Complementary Medicine, *June 2000*

periods, the discomfort in her lower back ("Is it my ovaries or my kidneys?") and a strange discharge from her nipple. She describes feeling desperate for energy, which she is greatly lacking.

Joanne appears quite anxious about her health complaints. She describes herself as "on the anxious neurotic side but positive." She has controlled her health through her diet but only a slight error produces profound repercussions. "If I eat an allergic food I get gas, bloating, and diarrhea. When asked about her fears she offers: "I am afraid of health things and things about business—am I going to make it? I begin to have panic about that. I can get diarrhea from being too emotional, too!"

As Joanne elaborates about her nature, she says, "I am a perfectionist. I get stuck in a quagmire and I can't think."

I ask about her marriage and Joanne admits some regret about not having children. "I wanted him to be the one to say 'let's have children!' I didn't want to make it a huge issue in my life so I chose career. I've got to achieve something."

Joanne was given Argentum Nitricum, or homeopathic silver nitrate.

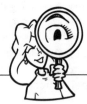

Curious Clues

People who benefit from Argentum Nitricum usually have strong issues around performance (as do all the metal remedies), often feeling that the love and attention they received from their parents was conditional on what they did instead of who they were. In addition, the remedy was chosen for the following:

➤ Diarrhea after eating

➤ Diarrhea from emotions

➤ Anxiety about health, fear of impending disease

➤ Fear of failure

➤ Fear of insanity (in this case Alzheimer's)

➤ Confusion of mind

Joanne returned in one month with a very positive report. "I am a lot better. I feel more attuned and balanced. I got better in a few days, especially my gastrointestinal tract. I still have to be careful what I eat but not as bad as it was. Mentally and emotionally I've been pretty darn good! I know before I was talking about being depressed, hormonal stuff, having a hard time at work. I have been happy and am back to enjoying my work again."

Joanne has continued to improve with occasional doses of Argentum Nitricum.

Irritable Bowel Syndrome

Having a condition known as IBS (irritable bowel syndrome) usually creates some tension due to the mayhem after mealtime. This is the most common digestive disorder affecting one of five adults in America, with twice as many women as men. There is no known cause for the cramping pain, gassiness, bloating, constipation and/or diarrhea that are often associated with IBS. Pain is often brought on by eating and relieved by a bowel movement. The food link is often very strong; it's typical that IBS patients are nervous around mealtime, which tends to also aggravate this condition. Many patients have shared this disappointment, having to decline invitations to social events, travel, or fully relax at family functions.

Common triggers for IBS include stress; food intolerances such as high-fat content, chocolate, milk products, alcohol, caffeine; and reproductive hormones.

Though diagnosis is important to rule out other conditions, conventional medicines are designed to be supportive since the origin of IBS is unknown. Antispasmodic and antidepressant drugs are used, but discouraged if the patient becomes dependent on them. I have found that homeopathy can be an enormous relief for sufferers of IBS, cutting down on both the symptoms and the constellation of concerns that often accompany this irritable situation. I hope the next patient's story gives you a clear example of homeopathic help that awaits you.

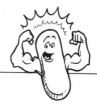

Potent Pellets

A new study suggests a person's emotional and mental state may have an effect on your digestive system. Researchers tested the effects using emotional words and found that between 70 percent and 77 percent of the time muscles responded by either relaxing or contracting. These findings suggest a closer link between the mind and your gut.

Source: Digestive Diseases and Sciences, June 2000

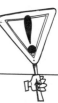

Caution Keeper

A popular new treatment for irritable bowel syndrome (IBS) could cause severe intestinal side effects. The FDA recently ordered Glaxo Wellcome, Inc., to attach to every bottle of Lotronex a plain-speaking pamphlet explaining the risks. This medicine is prescribed to women with IBS whose main symptom is diarrhea. It doesn't work for men.

Source: Associated Press, 2000

IBS: Tormented Talent

"As a child, I remember being so excited that I'd have an upset stomach. I'd internal-ize things." This was Todd, who came in for treatment of irritable bowel syndrome (IBS). As a musician, Todd was particularly tormented by the uncertain cramping and diarrhea that may take him out of work at a moment's notice. "If I'm not given the proper respect or given undue criticism, then I'm quick to anger, but I hold it in. I set the bar pretty high at work and in my relationships. If I get less respect from those around me, I feel like I'm less of a man, and I'll get angry inside."

Todd had been in the music business for over 20 years, but complained that he'd never really made a success of himself like he thought he should have. "I have a lot of issues around succeeding. I won't participate in a project if I feel others are much better than I am. I have piles of unfinished projects. I just can't share them with oth-ers. I don't feel comfortable telling people what to do, even though I know. I share the leadership roles."

Todd experienced the typical cramping, abdominal pain, and intestinal gas, which were relieved by his bowel movements. He noticed that nerves affected his intestines and wanted a better solution than taking medication. He continued through the visit expressing great ideas, but being doubtful about the projects and his own self worth. "I may look great to others, but my self-esteem is poor most of the time; other times I believe I've got it together. I'm a perfectionist, but I can't let it out to others. I feel it's just not right, they wouldn't understand." I gave Todd Niobium.

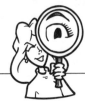

Curious Clues

Other signs of a person who would benefit from Niobium include ...

➤ Abdominal pains with diarrhea.

➤ Doubt whether they are special.

➤ Indecisive whether they will exert their influence.

➤ Unrealistic ideas about their creations.

➤ Evading their talents.

➤ Tormented by ambition.

➤ Tormented by not showing their talents.

Source: Scholten, 1996

Niobium is taken from the name Niobe the Greek daughter of Tantalus who was punished for her pride. What stuck out to me most in this case is Todd's true talent and ability with a layer of haughty pride. This prevents him from believing in himself or sharing his ideas with others. I believe there is a lack of realistic perception about himself and his work. Somewhere in there is Todd; he's not been able to "find himself" and continues to struggle with doubt.

Todd's IBS improved over the next couple of months. He was also able to relax around the issues of his talent and begin to share more of his projects with others. This helped his professional life and relationships. These seemed intimately tied to his IBS. As his professional life improved, so did his IBS. This took a number of months, but the lasting results, through ups and downs in his career, have not increased his gastric symptoms.

Homeopaths specialize in finding the individual symptoms among the common complaints of these gastric glitches. The safe, nontoxic approach that homeopathy offers can bring about the lasting relief you've just read about.

The Least You Need to Know

➤ Homeopathic help is available for many digestive complaints.

➤ Heartburn affects nearly 60 million Americans annually.

➤ Lack of exercise, adequate fluids, and fiber often contribute to chronic constipation.

➤ Calcaria Silicate may help individuals who are constipated with hard stools and have timid, withdrawn personalities.

➤ A recent study showed homeopathy and proper fluids to be effective in 85 percent of the children studied with acute diarrhea, the number-one killer of children in the world.

➤ Homeopathic treatments for irritable bowel syndrome include helping the debilitating symptoms and improving stability.

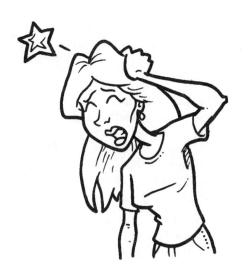

Chapter 19

Purging Your Pain

In This Chapter

➤ Healing headaches with homeopathy

➤ Learn valuable tips on treatments for nagging bursitis

➤ Take the ache out of arthritis using the effective diluted solutions of homeopathy

➤ Let homeopathy negate the never-ending nerve pain of sciatica

---

Pain can be such a drain that by the end of the day you're exhausted both physically and emotionally. Persistent pain makes it difficult to concentrate at work and limits your family fun. We've probably all known pain caused by accidental bumps and bruises. Perhaps you've even healed from a serious injury, but what if you had a painful partner every day of your life that seemed to run the show. You may or may not make plans to go out with friends, go for a hike, or play catch with your grand-children depending on your level of pain.

Learn valuable homeopathic solutions that others have chosen to gain freedom from pain. I'll be discussing safe and effective treatment options for headaches, bursitis, arthritis, and sciatica.

Headaches: Trouble in the Tower

Pounding, bursting, throbbing are all words we use to describe the horrors of head-aches. According to the American Council for Headache Education, over 50 million Americans experience some form of severe headache. About 26 million of us have

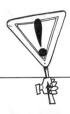

Caution Keeper

If you suffer from chronic headaches, watch your reactions to these common food triggers and additives: wheat, chocolate, monosodium glutamate (MSG), hot dogs, luncheon meats, alcohol, sulfites, vinegar, and nuts.

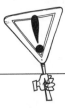

Caution Keeper

Nonsteroidal anti-inflammatory drugs (NSAIDS) are a common medication for mild to moderate pain. Check with your doctor or pharmacist for possible drug interactions with other medications that you may be taking such as methotrexate and ketoprofen.

migraine headaches, either with an aura (classic migraine) or without (common migraine). Severe debilitating recurring headaches pound about one million Americans down per year.

Headaches can be the primary condition or a symptom of an underlying situation such as high blood pressure, glaucoma, sinusitis, or less likely cerebral tumors or meningitis. Thorough diagnosis is the first part of a good treatment plan, and conventional medicine offers pain-killing analgesics including acetaminophen, NSAIDS, or opioid narcotics.

Homeopathic care takes your diagnosis and finds the remedy that matches your overall health picture, paying close attention to those individual characteristics that are unique to you. Take a look at the next patient's headache history and the homeopathic medicine that helped to end the pain.

Chronic Headaches (Presented by Savitri Clarke)

Helen is a 54-year-old woman who suffers from chronic severe headaches. As we walk into the consultation room, she looks down and has trouble making eye contact, appearing embarrassed or even ashamed. She has had many losses in her life including a divorce with two young children at home, and the death of her grandson and son-in-law from drowning a year before. She appears weighted down and unhappy. "I feel like I don't have any blood running through my veins. The headaches hurt so bad. I feel cold. I don't know why I get them, I can't think straight when I have a headache and when they finally go away I feel so drained. It feels like my head is going to explode. Even my teeth hurt. I feel sick to my stomach with them. It helps if I press on my temples really hard. I am getting hot flashes now, too. Never had them before. I've been depressed my whole life. My cup is always half empty. I back down from confrontation and I am afraid for anyone to be angry with me."

Helen grew up with a mother who was constantly yelling at her and telling her she was stupid. Her father was also very dictatorial and demanding. No one ever talked about their feelings, leaving her feeling emotionally repressed.

"This is what it must feel like to be dead, nothing is moving or circulating inside. With the hot flashes, the body is cold but I am very hot."

Helen has had headaches most of her life. They were better after she got married and had children but returned with a vengeance with menopause five years ago. She suffered the deaths of her grandson and son-in-law silently. Now she takes care of her very ill mother who lives upstairs and is endlessly needy without showing any gratitude. "I am very stressed and I don't sleep well. I don't know when she is going to bang her cane and I want to make sure I hear her. It is such a big responsibility. I feel trapped more than ever now."

Helen was given the remedy Magnesium Muriaticum, which is homeopathic magnesium chloride.

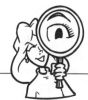

Curious Clues

Magnesium Muriaticum is known as a remedy for orphans who were abandoned, never receiving the love and affection they deserved. These individuals feel hurt but must not show this and remain independent to defend themselves from further disappointment. It was chosen on the following indications:

➤ Headaches; hard pressure

➤ History of chronic headaches

➤ Sensation of internal heat with external cold

➤ Fear of confrontation and people getting angry

➤ History of lack of nurturance as a child (forsaken), feeling unlovable

➤ Repressed emotions

➤ Overly responsible

Helen returned two months later reporting, "The headaches are much better. My mother still aggravates me but I don't hold onto that aggravation. I just let it go now. My cup is more full now."

Over the next three years, Helen's headaches completely disappeared. Helen needed only three more doses of her remedy, the last one when her mother was dying. After repeating the remedy, she wrote saying, "Thank you so very much. I would never have been able to get through the death of my mother without the help of homeopathy." She has been well since and remains free of headaches and depression.

Bursitis: Pain on the Point

Bursitis is an inflammation of the bursa, which are the saclike capsules that surround many joints such as elbows, knees, or hips. These small sacs are located between tendons and bones to help your muscles move by cushioning them against friction. When the bursa is inflamed, every motion seems to have the characteristic persistent dull ache.

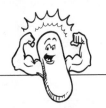

Potent Pellets

Bursitis has been bothering workers for a long time. The occupations usually match the malady's name as in policeman's heel, housemaid's knee, miner's beat shoulder, or weaver's bottom.

Overuse is often the beginning of bursitis; redness, swelling, and pain soon follow with motion making the dull pain worse. Tendinitis affects the soft tissue that connects bone to muscle. This often has sharper pains and is not accompanied by swelling and fluid accumulation as in bursitis. Conventional medicine recommends corticosteroid injections or, more rarely, surgical removal or large-needle aspiration for chronic bursitis. As you will see with the next patient's story, homeopathic treatment seeks to reduce pain and improve overall health while eliminating the need for conventional therapy or medication.

Chronic Bursitis: The Bearcat Bursa

"Both shoulders hurt again, and you better get on it. It hurts like a bastard." Sammy had chronic bursitis in both shoulders with intermittent pain for about two decades. He used to run a local catering business, a hot spot in the community for years. "Nobody could touch us. We were the best and everybody knew it."

Sammy was all business. He always came 15 to 20 minutes early before his appointment saying that he would like to get in early, because he had so much to do. He was nervous to get going, even when we were ahead of schedule. He was retired now, but you'd never know it by his pace; lots of business meetings. "I got a lot going on. I love the action, you know."

Sammy had a lot of scores to settle with his family and many business acquaintances over the years. He never let go of them. He'd rail about how they cheated him, and he would like to go "break both their kneecaps."

Sammy had a history of psoriasis with dry thick-crusted skin, gout, and pneumonia. He has been a heavy drinker for years but was cutting back now. His chronic bursitis is always better with rest and worse with even the slightest motion, making it difficult for him to sleep at night. The winter cold is challenging for his bursitis, and he has a tendency to get bronchitis. I gave Sammy Bryonia Alba.

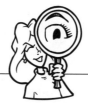

Curious Clues

White Bryony, or *Bryonia Alba*, is the fast-growing perennial plant from northern and southeastern Europe. Pain with motion is a common bursitis symptom, but Sammy's symptoms that were aggravated by cold, business-like priorities, and psoriasis with impatience started me thinking about Bryonia Alba. Other signs that gave me confidence to prescribe included ...

➤ Anxiety, compelled to do something.

➤ Talks of business.

➤ Dry skin eruptions, thick patches.

➤ Obstinate, headstrong, threatening.

➤ Pain and coughs worse from cold.

➤ Pain worse from even the slightest motion.

➤ Alcohol abuse.

➤ Gout.

➤ Discontented, dissatisfied, displeased.

Sammy's bursitis pain was helped within a few days. He had better motion with less pain. Over the next few months, his psoriasis greatly improved during the winter when it is usually worse. His other aches and pains improved, as did his overall energy level. His daughter said he was less standoffish and easier to be with. He has continued to feel good, getting off all his medications and has only needed Bryonia Alba occasionally for actively-related flare-ups. He has felt good for the last six years.

Arthritis: Snap, Crackle, and Pop

If you are one of the 50 million Americans who suffer from one of more than 100 forms of arthritis, then you know how painful this condition can be. When they work properly, our joints can provide great flexibility and ease of movement. When the pain, inflammation, stiffness, or even deformity begins in one or more joints, the ease will seize, the joints can freeze, and we begin to plead for some help!

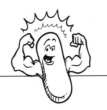

Half of all people over age 65 have some form of arthritis. The smooth layer of tissue or cartilage that covers the bones or the fluid-filled capsules of joints become disturbed by genetics, disease, or overwork. Then you will feel the pain and restriction of motion that often characterizes arthritis.

Types of Arthritis

Patients often describe arthritic joints like "that hip's bothering me again!" as if it were a separate bothersome neighbor that causes trouble occasionally. While there are still forms of arthritis that are not fully understood, here's a rundown of the different types of arthritis we have some understanding about …

➤ **Osteoarthritis.** Average age at onset: over 40. Characteristics: gradual stiffness and pain, enlargement of the joint.

➤ **Rheumatoid arthritis.** Average age at onset: between 25 and 50. Characteristics: autoimmune condition (immune system cells kill body cells), inflammation of the joint and neighboring tendons, muscles, and nerves.

➤ **Spondyloarthropathies.** Average age at onset: from 20 to 40. Characterisitics: spinal inflammation and pain, often causing postural changes.

➤ **Gout.** Average age at onset: from 40 to 43. Characteristics: sudden severe pain and swelling of a large joint, usually the big toe.

➤ **Lupus.** Average age at onset: from 18 to 50. Characteristics: fever, weakness, facial and joint pain.

➤ **Juvenile rheumatoid arthritis.** Average age at onset: under 18. Characteristics: Autoimmune condition, stiffness often in the knees, wrists, or hands. May involve kidneys, heart, lungs, and nervous system.

➤ **Infectious arthritis.** Average age at onset: any. Characteristics: body aches, chills, fever, low blood pressure, swelling and pain that spreads to other joints.

➤ **Kawasaki syndrome.** Average age at onset: six months to 11 years. Characteristics: fever, joint pain, and rash on palms and soles, heart problems.

Conventional medical treatment of arthritis ranges from over-the-counter painkillers and topical analgesics to gold compounds, corticosteriods, or immunosuppressive drugs for more severe autoimmune arthritis. Potential for serious side effects exists, so communication and monitoring with your physician is advisable. Homeopathic treatment seeks to ease the burden you feel on your joints while reducing the tendency for your body to produce arthritic symptoms. This nontoxic, nonhabit-forming therapy can be exceptionally effective and assist your body in life-changing healing as you'll read in the next patient's story.

Rheumatoid Arthritis (Presented by Savitri Clarke)

Johnny is a somewhat overweight 13-year-old boy who walks stiffly into the consulting room. He immediately starts making jokes, saying he is trying to make this as interesting as possible and complains that his friends have grown out of having fun. He says the pain started two years ago. "While playing soccer I began having trouble with my feet. Now I go out and exercise, have fun, play tennis, then come home and watch TV. The next time I want to stand it really hurts: knees, ankles, feet. It's a struggle to move, especially going up stairs. Hot baths help. I ache more after swimming in cold water."

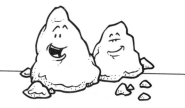

Natural Nuggets

A pineapple a day may keep arthritis away! Fresh pineapple contains the enzyme bromelain, which can be used to reduce inflammation. Freezing can destroy the enzyme, so make sure it's fresh for best results.

Johnny is a personable young man and fun to be with. He seems to have some anxiety and seems concerned with what impression he is making. He has been on many medications, which either helped very little or made him depressed. He has a history of chronic ear infections—32 in all—then got ear tubes, which stopped the recurrent infections. I asked Johnny what was happening in his life when the pain started. He was not happy when his parents decided to divorce and cried a lot. Then his mother started seeing someone. "There was discussion of me, my sister, and mom moving into her boyfriend's house. I was nervous about it. I felt everything was changing and I was anxious and depressed. I thought I would have to bond with my mom's boyfriend's kids. I don't like to meet new people. I didn't want to have to live around these people. I felt uncomfortable when we moved in with them."

I asked about other anxieties Johnny might have. He said he has had lots. "I was afraid of cats and dogs. I was afraid of loud noises, of someone blasting a radio in a car. I was afraid of eating at other's houses; afraid they poisoned the food, at least that was my excuse. I think it was more about being observed, about the way I was eating. Last summer I became very freaked out about bugs; afraid they will crawl on me, I guess. I can't go to sleep if bugs are in my room."

When asked about his nature, Johnny said, "I am a nice person. I am afraid of being embarrassed. If my teacher calls on me in class and I don't know the answer I will be humiliated. Don't want the teachers making a fool out of me. One of my teachers screams at you if you don't know the answer. I panic. I don't know if he is going to scream at me."

Johnny's mother describes him as an anxious newborn who cried a lot. He had trouble separating from Mom to enter school. There was a bully at preschool and every morning he cried to stay with Mom. But he thinks it had more to do with separation anxiety than the bully.

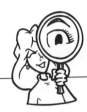

Curious Clues

In addition to the previous characteristics, Johnny was given Calcaria Carbonica because he had ...

➤ Joint pain that was alleviated by warmth.

➤ Joint pain that was exacerbated after rest.

➤ A history of many fears in childhood.

➤ A history of chronic ear infections.

➤ Using jesting, often as a way to alleviate their social anxiety.

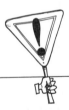

Caution Keeper

You put five times the body weight on your low back when sitting rather than standing. It's no wonder why further compression of the sciatic nerve by sitting on a toilet, riding in a car, or sitting on a bicycle seat tends to increase your pain.

He is very chilly and prefers warm weather.

Johnny was given Calcaria Carbonica, homeopathic calcium carbonate. This remedy comes from the oyster shell and the main feeling of people who benefit from this remedy is the need for stability and security. Like the oyster without a shell, they seek protection. Therefore anything that threatens that security will cause great fear. Home is very important to this remedy type as they feel most secure there. There is great anxiety about how they appear to others.

When Johnny came back six weeks later, he was quite happy. "I am able to do a lot of physical activities without being crippled the next day." His feet still get sore if he walks for a long time but he recovers much quicker than before. His mother says, "Most noticeably his whole affect is better. He is more cheerful and optimistic and upbeat. His whole attitude about things in general is much better."

Over the next six months, Johnny's arthritis symptoms totally disappeared. His fears were greatly reduced, including his fear of bugs. He said "I don't care about the bugs; it's not much of an issue anymore."

Johnny can now run a couple of miles with no pain during or after. He is even on the soccer team now and has no discomfort.

Sciatica: The Nagging Nerve

A pain in the butt is literally what you get with sciatica. Plus the burning or numbness that shoots down the back or side of your legs to the ankles or toes. Sciatica is usually one-sided, and its pain is present when you sit, stand, or even lie down. The term is commonly given to a pain caused by compression of the sciatic nerve that runs from the middle of your butt to the toes. The pressure can be caused from herniated or slipped disks in your lower spine, muscle spasms in the low back or hip (sacroiliac or piriformis), or more rarely an intraspinal tumor. Getting a thorough diagnosis will ensure the best chance at appropriate and effective treatment.

Conventional medicines include muscle relaxers or corticosteroid injection near the site of pain. My patients are often counseled to modify running, bicycling, or any activity that increases pain. Stretching exercises are a favorite of mine, with a home program as your ticket to freedom from pain.

I have used homeopathy in both acute and chronic cases with good results. Take a look at the next patient's story and see why it was essential that she chose a nontoxic treatment to help her with sciatica.

Pregnancy-Induced Sciatica (Presented by Savitri Clarke)

Christy was six months pregnant when she came for help with very painful sciatica. Her pregnancy was going well. But she complained of severe pain in her right buttock radiating down the side of her leg. The pain was better walking and with a warm bath and worse sitting or lying, especially lying on the right side. It was affecting her sleep and making her life much more difficult.

When I asked about her spirits she said, "I get irritated with the way people deal with their kids. I overreact. I expect people to do something and they don't. I am intolerant of rigid perfection in people. I don't yell, instead I suppress my anger so that I feel so irritable all the time. I even wake up irritable!" When I questioned what other things aggravated her in general, she offered, "I get more irritable when I am hungry and tired. When I am hungry I must eat right away or I get very impatient and irritable."

I wanted to give Christy some relief because I knew this condition would only get worse as her pregnancy and weight gain progressed. She received Lycopodium, or homeopathic club moss.

Since Christy had all of these symptoms, I expected she would do well. She called in a week to say that the sciatica pain was down to an occasional twinge. Over the next 10 days it disappeared entirely and Christy was able to complete her pregnancy and birth her baby without this gnawing pain.

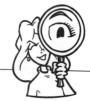

Curious Clues

Lycopodium is a remedy that is very useful for right-sided musculo-skeletal problems, especially when they are improved by motion and warm bathing. Sciatica that is made worse by lying on the painful side is another indication. In addition, Lycopodium is helpful when suppressed anger comes out in irritability and when there is irritability on waking, when hungry, or when tired.

Pain often can prevent us from enjoying life more fully. It forces its way into our lives with severe disruption to our lifestyle. As you have read, homeopathic care may be the option you've been seeking for lasting relief and overall improvement of health.

The Least You Need to Know

➤ Homeopathic treatment may be a viable option for some of the 50 million Americans who suffer from severe headaches.

➤ Magnesium Muriaticum is helpful for people with chronic headaches, with personality traits that include being overly responsible, repressed emotions, and feelings of being unloved.

➤ Bursitis that is worse from even the slightest movement, with an obstinate, business-like individual, may benefit from the homeopathic remedy Bryonia Alba.

➤ About 50 million Americans suffer from over 100 forms of arthritis; homeopathy may help.

➤ The sickening pain of sciatica is caused by pressure on the sciatic nerve, which runs from your backside to your toes.

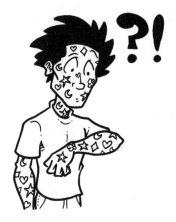

Chapter 20

Mysterious Maladies

In This Chapter

➤ Learn how homeopathy can help with the lingering symptoms of Lyme disease

➤ Forget your fibromyalgia pain and fatigue with the diluted solutions of homeopathy

➤ Discover the way homeopathy ends debilitating vertigo and the ringing and fullness in the ears with Ménière's disease

➤ Mono messing up your life? Get a tip for effective homeopathic treatment

---

There is much in life that's a mystery, and the practice of medicine is no exception. Despite tremendous advances of our technical and diagnostic capabilities, there are still many conditions that are not well understood. I've heard patients wish for a disease that was better understood or even recognized. Their frustration rises at trying to get a consensus from their team of medical providers regarding what's going on and what can they do about it. Unfortunately, some conditions are still shrouded in a mist of disbelief, misinformation, and confusion.

Homeopathy, which began in an age of medical uncertainty and harsh treatments, has been sifting through the symptoms of suffering for more than 200 years. This chapter will show how this medical art deals with such conditions as Lyme disease and Ménière's disease. We'll also take a look at the often debilitating conditions of mononucleosis and fibromyalgia and illuminate the homeopathic approaches that I've found to be safe and effective. In these cases, successful homeopathic outcomes are often referred to as magical or miraculous. I can assure you it's the same sound, principled prescribing that you've read about throughout this book. Have fun finding solutions through the fog for some of medicine's difficult dilemmas.

Lyme Disease: Getting Ticked Off

The great outdoors can have some very great risks if you are part of the more than 99,000 cases of Lyme disease that have been reported to the Centers for Disease Control and Prevention (CDC) from 1982 to 1996. Experts believe that number may be under-reported by as much as 10 times.

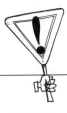

Caution Keeper

Approximately 15 percent to 30 percent of Lyme disease cases show no early symptoms such as the characteristic round red rash. If allowed to progress to late-stage Lyme disease, bacteria can affect joints, tendons, your heart, or your nervous system, resulting in permanent damage.

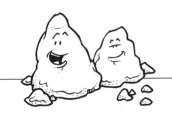

Natural Nuggets

If you find a tick attached, use a pair of tweezers to grab it close to your skin and pull straight out. Do not twist or crush the tick, because it could inject more bacteria into you. Keep the tick and show it to your health-care provider for correct identification. Watch the area closely for about three weeks for signs of a rash.

Lyme disease was given its name in 1975 because of the close clustering of cases in Lyme, Connecticut. It has since been reported in 49 states, but more than 90 percent of all cases develop in Massachusetts to Maryland, in Wisconsin, Minnesota, California, and Oregon. Lyme disease is the most commonly reported tick-borne illness in the United States.

Most patients are children and young adults who live or play in heavily wooded areas. Ticks originally live on mice, deer, rats, dogs, cats, horses, and even birds. They fall off their first ride into brush or woods and wait to hitchhike on you or your pet as you pass by. Ticks are small and hard to spot. They will painlessly bite you, and then feed on your blood for several days. If it's infected by Lyme disease, then so are you. The longer the tick is attached, the greater the risk of developing Lyme disease.

Treatment with conventional medicine involves the use of antibiotics, which is highly effective when the disease is caught early. I always suggest to patients that they receive antibiotic treatment for suspected Lyme disease. The late-stage Lyme disease which you'll read about in the next patient's story is how homeopathic treatment is typically used. You will see how homeopathic care can be of great relief for this serious condition.

Late-Stage Lyme Disease (Presented by Savitri Clarke)

Carol is an active 73-year-old drama teacher and consultant. She is warm and charming and easy to talk to. Four months ago, while visiting her daughter, she started feeling odd. She had a fever for three days and a big oval-shaped rash in her inner thigh with a little spot in the middle. She never saw the tick. "I had been pushing myself harder than normal getting ready for my daughter's wedding. I wanted to make the garden pretty so she would like it."

Carol took antibiotics for a month. She got through the wedding and thought it would all just go away. But she was mistaken. Over the next two months she suffered with severe sore muscles. It started in her head and spread to her face, shoulders, arms, and inner thighs. All her joints were stiff, especially her knees. She "felt like an old lady." She began having low-grade fevers at night with chills and sweats. Her physician ran tests to rule out a brain tumor, leukemia, and tuberculosis. Since then she has much lower energy and wakes up very stiff every morning. A hot shower feels good and makes a big difference.

When asked about her nature she said, "I spend time not wanting to make other people unhappy. I had a theory if I was so positive in my attitude, I could get rid of the Lyme, but it is still there. My brother raises his voice, and I feel 'you jerk,' but the way of dealing with it is not to get angry. I just want to be liked. I get upset with myself when I have sustained anger about something. I never get angry with my family."

"Instead of just going out and dealing with it, I avoid it." When Carol was little, it upset her when her parents would fight. "I just wanted them to be happy." I gave her Magnesium Sulphuricum.

After one month Carol reported that she had had some itchy skin eruptions for the first couple of weeks, which had subsided. "My stiffness is better and no recurrence of fever and sweats. I started exercising on the bike for the first time. My arms are still weak but getting better." Over the next year, Carol saw a return to her old energetic self with the post-Lyme stiffness disappearing.

Fibromyalgia: A Tussle with Your Muscle

Fibro (fiber) and myalgia (muscle pain) characterizes this often-devastating chronic rheumatic pain disorder of unknown cause. The pain is usually described as "achy," but a few patients tell me they can also experience burning, throbbing, stabbing, or shooting pain. To make this dish sound even more unappetizing, fibromyalgia is often accompanied by

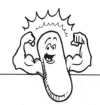

Potent Pellets

Doctors may be able to determine much more quickly whether a patient has Lyme disease. A new test identifies immune system clusters in about a week, while the standard test detects only antibodies, which can take up to several weeks.

Source: Journal of the American Medical Association (JAMA), November 24, 1995

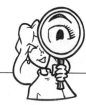

Curious Clues

Carol is warm-blooded and has a tendency to skin eruptions, both signs of the remedy Sulphur. I knew she needed a remedy in the Magnesium family, because of her aversion to conflict and her great need to please and be liked. I chose Magnesium Sulphuricum, homeopathic magnesium sulphate.

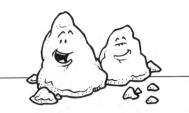

Natural Nuggets

Studies on patients with fibromyalgia have shown there is inefficient use of oxygen in the muscles. Mild to moderate exercise that's built up slowly over time can benefit the oxygen-starved muscle tissues, while high-intensity workouts usually cause more harm than good. Check with your health-care provider or a qualified personal trainer for a safe program.

side orders of chronic headaches, strange skin sensations, temporomandibular joint pain (TMJ), insomnia, irritable bowel syndrome (IBS), anxiety, palpitations, fatigue, poor memory, painful menstruation, and depression. Diagnosis is difficult because we don't know why people get this condition. Patients are often frustrated because they have met many physicians who say, "It's all in your head." There have been links to the onset of symptoms and Epstein-Barr virus (EBV) that causes mononucleosis. Since pain and fatigue are key symptoms, others have thought it may be connected to chronic fatigue immune deficiency syndrome (CFIDS).

Fibromyalgia occurs mostly in women, many who have experienced insomnia, anxiety, stress, or depression. The symptoms are often severe enough to greatly interrupt their normal life and in many cases, patients are unable to stay at work or maintain normal household activities such as cooking, child care, or shopping.

The Painful Points of Fibromyalgia

Fibromyalgia is often challenging to properly diagnose because of the many overlapping symptoms it has in common with other conditions. There are nine sets of diagnostic trigger points that are typically tender to the touch.

The tender points used to diagnose fibromyalgia are …

➤ Around the lower neck.

➤ Upper chest by the second rib.

➤ Around the upper thigh.

➤ Middle of the knee joint.

➤ Base of the skull.

➤ Neck and upper back.

➤ Midback.

➤ Inside of the elbow.

➤ Upper and outer muscles of the buttocks.

Conventional treatment of fibromyalgia depends on the symptoms and may combine several drugs including low-dose tricyclic antidepressants, aspirin, NSAIDS, lidocaine

injections, or a seratonin-specific re-uptake in-
hibitor. Massage, stretching, exercise, and acupuncture have also been recommended by myself and
others for relief. Patience and consistency are
important in this condition. Gaining back quality
sleep and managing your emotions are also key
goals for your homeopathic care. I hope the next
patient's story will aid your understanding of the
long-lasting solutions available for you with homeopathy.

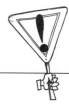

Caution Keeper

Saturated fats interfere with
circulation as well as raise choles-
terol. If you suffer from fibromyalgia, avoid eating meats and
diary products, which are high in
fat, because they also promote
inflammatory response and
increased pain.

Fibromyalgia: The Work Horse Hurts

"I'm goal-oriented," said Sarah. "I've got to get it
done. My family calls me to fix it and then I'm on
the job. If I can't meet the goal, I'm stressed. I'll
stay up till midnight during the week polishing
woodwork if it's on my to-do list."

Sarah had come into my office for treatment related to fibromyalgia/chronic fatigue
immune deficiency syndrome (CFIDS). She was a 32-year-old married woman who
began to experience ongoing fatigue and increasingly severe pain in her neck, back,
chest, and legs. This greatly interfered with her busy lifestyle and the plans she
had for herself. She had just started a new job, was remodeling her home with her
husband, getting her Master's degree, and preparing for family holidays.

When I asked her what it was like for her growing up, she shared, "As a child, my father always told me I wasn't good enough. We were not allowed to have emotions
show. My father is still alive. I have flashbacks now and that makes me sick and
angry. I forgive him, but have not forgotten the words he spoke. I guess I still hold a
lot in."

I asked her how she managed to be so busy. "I have an order to do things. I'd never
think of doing things out of order. I used to get anxiety attacks if I couldn't do my list
or housework in a particular order."

She went on to say that she is praised at her job for being organized and accomplished, but even her bosses tell her to take it easy. She is exhausted and hurts all
over, but pushes through it all to get to her goals. If she does not bake a cake and
make a homemade gift for someone's birthday, she feels guilty, like she hasn't tried
hard enough. She will work into the night finishing the lists she creates. Spastic
muscle pain and anxiety frequently keep her from having a good night's sleep. I gave
Sarah Ferrum Metallicum.

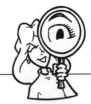

Curious Clues

The extreme levels of organizing and hard work to push to a goal led me to the Ferrum series of homeopathic remedies. I originally gave Sarah Ferrum Nitricum because of the tension created by over-assertiveness. This was only partially effective. Ferrum Metallicum or iron is a hard-working metal and has given her lasting results. Here are some themes of Ferrum that I matched with Sarah's situation:

➤ Persevering in your job

➤ Persistence in your tasks, toughness

➤ Perfectionism

➤ Order, rules, routine

➤ Failure of task turns to guilt

➤ Struggling to push through obstacles

➤ Insomnia, sleeplessness

➤ Joint and muscle pain

Sarah returned for a six-week follow-up and was still a busy bee, but noted that her muscle pain was much better, and her energy was more stable. "I'm energized, but it's a more steady pace. I don't have to push myself as much. My father doesn't like to talk to me, but now I'm content with having him just listen to what I've got to say."

Several months passed, and Sarah's fibromyalgia and CFIDS symptoms continued to decrease. Muscle spasms were hardly noticed, and she has generally been feeling good. She has begun to ask for help from co-workers so she doesn't have to stay late at her job. She continues to be aware of doing too much, can now leave things undone, is taking time to sleep, and is enjoying a renewed relationship with her husband. That was four years ago and Sarah continues to cut back and still amaze us all!

Ménière's Disease: Inner Fear of Your Ear

The cause of Ménière's disease, named after the French physician P. Ménière (1799–1862) who first described it, is unknown and the predictability of when symptoms begin is also in question. This disguised disorder is characterized by recurrent severe *vertigo,* hearing loss, ringing in the ears, and a feeling of fullness like there's water in your ear all the time.

Attacks of vertigo may appear suddenly and last from a couple of hours to an entire day. This dizzying disorder is usually accompanied by nausea and vomiting. Typically only one ear is affected, but in 10 percent to 15 percent of unlucky patients, both ears can be involved.

Treatment with conventional medicine varies since a clear cause is difficult to determine. Medications for tinnitus and vertigo are given to control symptoms, and surgery is recommended for severely disabled patients.

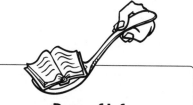

Dose of Info

Like a continuous carnival ride, **vertigo** is dizziness, a sensation of whirling motion, either of oneself or of external objects. You're not sure whether you or the rooms are spinning.

This is an area where homeopathy has the potential to shine. It's a safe, nontoxic approach, will cause no harm, and has the possibility of helping a patient whose options are limited. The next patient's story will show you the value of investigating a homeopathic approach to healing.

Ménière's Disease (Presented by Savitri Clarke)

Terry is hoping to get help for her sudden attacks of severe dizziness, nausea, and ringing in her ears. When she arrives for her appointment she seems reluctant about revealing information about herself. "My symptoms began with a strange claustrophobic feeling and ringing in my ears four years ago. At that time I was going through menopause and also had begun taking estrogen replacement therapy. Then I started having severe episodes. I would suddenly become disoriented, couldn't walk, my balance was completely off, and I had to touch the wall so as not to fall. I couldn't focus my eyes. The internal dizziness makes me start to vomit violently. This goes on for about 24 hours."

Terry talks about how debilitating these episodes are. She must stay in bed. There is nothing she can take or do, just suffer through it. She continues, "I am a classroom teacher. I don't know what creates the most anxiety for me: wondering whether it is going to happen or the volume of the ringing in my ears."

When asked about her nature, she shared, "I demand perfection of myself at home and at school. I have set high standards of myself. Being a good mother was very important for me. I never allow myself much downtime. Time is to be used, not for being idle." Then Terry described how upset she was when her only son attempted suicide. He later admitted that he was gay. This was very disappointing for Terry and she blamed herself. "What did we do to this child that made him so unhappy?" Terry received Kali Muriaticum, homeopathic potassium chloride.

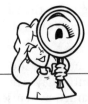

Curious Clues

Kali Muriaticum is a remedy for a woman who feels a strong duty to be a good mother and take care of her family. They often learn this from being the eldest daughter who must take care of their younger brothers and sisters. Her feeling of having failed with her son was what most likely weakened her constitutionally. In addition, Terry had the following symptoms of Kali Muriaticum:

➤ Ménière's disease

➤ Noises in the ear with vertigo

➤ Sudden vomiting

➤ Incessant vomiting

Terry returned six weeks later saying, "I did very well. I still have some ringing in my ear but I have had no sensation of dizziness or any episodes. Even the ringing is better as the tone has stayed very low." Regarding her son, she has now realized, "I have to step back. I can't be the mother that makes it all right. My role is to continue to let him know I love him."

Over the next year, with a few doses of her remedy, Terry's Ménière's disease disappeared with only an occasional low ringing in her ears remaining.

Mononucleosis

When I was in junior high school, I was convinced that parents used *mononucleosis,* commonly called *mono,* as a scare tactic to curb our growing interest in kissing. Now I learn once again that Mom was right. Mono is so easy to get that 95 percent of people over the age of 35 have antibodies to mono in their blood, which means they've been infected by it. Most of us are infected in our childhood and symptoms are so mild they look like a common cold or flu. About 50 percent of children are infected by the age of five.

Mono is spread by close contact such as kissing, sharing food, drinks, or utensils, sexual contact, or through airborne carriers (as is the common cold virus).

Symptoms of Mono: Emphatic Lymphatics

Most people with mono feel better within two or three weeks. The incubation period or the time when you can infect others is about 10 days in children and 30 to 50 days in adults. When adolescents and adults contract mono, the symptoms can linger for a year or so with more mild recurring bouts of the outs (1 to 25 of all mono cases). Early symptoms of mono resemble the flu:

➤ Severe fatigue

➤ Headache

➤ Sore throat

➤ Chills and fever

➤ Muscle ache

After a day or two, you can add these to your experience:

➤ Swollen lymph nodes (neck, armpit, or groin)

➤ Jaundice (a yellow tinge to the skin and eyes)

➤ A measle-like rash anywhere on the face and body

➤ Tiny red spots or bruiselike areas inside the mouth

➤ Soreness in the upper-left abdomen (enlarged spleen)

Since there is no known cure for mono, conventional medical treatment is largely supportive, unless more serious complications develop. Homeopathic care seeks to bolster the tired immune system and aid you in a hasty recovery. Returning to the most complete state of health helps you stay strong so you avoid getting sick again. Read the next patient's story and discover how homeopathy managed the mono and more!

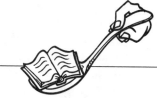

Dose of Info

Mononeucleous is an infectious viral disease. Most cases of mono are caused by the Epstein-Barr virus (EBV) and, more rarely, the cytomegalovirus (CMV); both are highly contagious and spread from person to person by close contact.

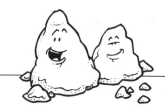

Natural Nuggets

A diagnosis of mono is made through a blood test called a heterophil antibody test. This will show Epstein-Barr virus–specific antibodies in the blood and confirm the presence of mononucleosis.

Infectious Mononucleosis (Presented by Savitri Clarke)

Ann had been a regular patient for several years. Thanks to homeopathy, she has seen her constant cough and asthmatic episodes almost totally eliminated. She is a sensitive eight-year-old child who seems to vibrate with excitement. Her generosity and caring for others is evident in her enjoyment of making special little gifts for people.

Ann has always felt fearful in crowded public places. Being so excitable, she can suffer from becoming overexcited when anticipating special events. She also can get very upset very quickly over little things.

Ann's mother brought her in one week after her diagnosis of mononucleosis. She had been having 104°F fevers around the clock for seven days. She had been taking Motrin every eight hours during this time but when it would wear off after about six hours. Then for the hour or two it took for the medicine to kick back in she was miserable. Ann said, "I am not bad now because I took medicine five hours ago. The worst part was last night. I couldn't move at all. My body was too heavy. I lost all my energy. I couldn't even talk. It was very painful; my muscles ached. I had a bad headache at the back of my head and a bad fever. When it starts up I feel shivering cold; then when I get hot I start writhing, getting hotter and hotter. Mom puts an ice pack on my head. I keep on going hot and cold. Then I take Motrin and it settles the fever."

Ann's mother adds that, "Last night was really bad. She couldn't talk; she was just laying there. We almost took her to the emergency room. She couldn't open her eyes, it just took too much strength." Then Ann remembers, "One strange thing was when my little sister closed the door to my room, I felt like I couldn't breathe. Like I would suffocate in there."

Ann was given one dose of Gelsemium, the yellow jasmine, with extra doses in case she should need it, and I asked Ann's mother to call me in 24 hours.

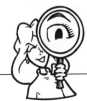

Curious Clues

I have treated many cases of the flu that looked like this. While this was a remedy I had never considered for Ann before, the symptoms of her mononucleosis clearly fit the Gelsemium picture:

➤ Severe chills alternating with heat

➤ Extreme weakness

➤ Great heaviness of the limbs, so heavy cannot walk

➤ Eyelids so heavy cannot open the eyes

➤ Severe muscle aches

➤ Occipital headache (base of skull)

➤ Feeling of suffocation, much better with open air

The next afternoon Ann's mother called me to say, "It was a miracle! She never got another fever! It was like the last dose of Motrin never wore off. She continued to feel fine and still does. She wanted to go to school this morning but I thought it best to wait one day to be sure she was okay." Ann never had another symptom of the mono and never even needed to repeat the remedy.

Gelsemium is a remedy for sensitive people who tend to experience hysteria over little things, with great fear in crowded public places, and great excitement and anxiety anticipating events. It is my belief that Ann's acute illness helped lead me to a deep constitutional remedy for her that will help her with her more chronic issues. This is often the case and is the reason why we pay close attention to the way our patients manifest their acute illnesses.

I believe that one of the strengths of homeopathic medicines is that they can be used as a valuable aid to healing even when the cause or conventional treatment of the condition is unclear or in question.

The Least You Need to Know

➤ About 15 percent to 30 percent of Lyme disease cases show no early warning symptoms such as a round red rash.

➤ Ferrum Metallicum can help fibromyalgia patients who show signs of extreme perfectionism, persistence, and live by order, rules, and routines.

➤ The persistent vomiting and noises in the ear of patients with Ménière's disease may be assisted by Kali Muriaticum.

➤ More than 50 percent of children have been infected by mononucleosis by the age of five; homeopathic medicines can be a valuable solution for the malady of mono.

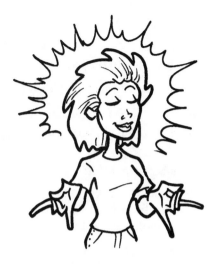

Healing from Within

Out of sight, out of mind? That may be dangerously true for the conditions we're about to discuss in this chapter. Without proper diagnosis and guidance, you may not be aware that you have diabetes or cancer. The symptoms you experience from these and other conditions such as a closed head injury and chronic fatigue might rule your life, but the cause may get by you. Without all the blood of a skull fracture, you might attribute how you feel to something else. You might even be given the line many people with chronic fatigue immune deficiency syndrome (CFIDS) hear, "It's all in your head."

Think seeing is believing? Tell that to someone who doesn't look any different, but gets up every day with the knowledge there is something terribly wrong going on inside. Through patients' stories, you'll see how homeopathy helps the symptoms and aids these individuals in achieving overall health and enjoyment of their life.

Diabetes: The Sugar Shutdown

An estimated 5.5 million Americans are being treated for diabetes, and researchers suggest there are another five million adults who don't even know they are diabetic.

There are two basic types of diabetes:

➤ **Diabetes insipidus (DI):** A temporary or chronic disorder of the neurohyprophyseal system due to a deficiency of the hormone vasopressin, characterized by excessive urination and thirst.

➤ **Diabetes mellitus (DM):** There are two types of diabetes mellitus:

Type I: Insulin dependent or juvenile diabetes, represents 10 percent to 15 percent of DM, usually diagnosed before age 30, genetically susceptible destruction of the beta cells, which produce insulin to help metabolize sugar in our bodies.

Type II: Noninsulin dependent, used to be called adult onset because most cases were being diagnosed over the age of 30, now a growing number of children and adolescents develop the characteristic nervousness and headaches of hypoglycemia.

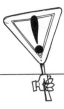

Caution Keeper

Undiagnosed diabetes has caused millions of people to lose their sight, and complications from diabetes is the third leading cause of death in the United States.

Source: The National Institutes of Health

Researchers of the human genome, the complete set of influential biological hereditary factors, believe that both Type I and II have a genetic link that runs in families. There are an estimated 20 million adults that have impaired glucose tolerance (IGT) who are at risk for developing diabetes.

You may not have any symptoms that you are aware of or you might brush it off as not a big deal. Type I (DM) children may begin to wet the bed when they had not previously. Irritability, frequent urination, abnormal thirst, nausea, vomiting, weakness, and weight loss are other signs to be cautious about. Type II (DM) is characterized by blurred vision, itching, increased thirst, fatigue, slow wound healing, and tingling or numbness in the feet. If you have any concerns about your condition, I suggest you see your health-care provider for a blood or urine test.

Experts agree that exercise and proper nutrition are highly important in managing the different forms of diabetes. I suggest getting educated on the selection of nutrients your body needs to function, and the treatment options and their risks that are available to you.

There is a wide range of insulin preparations available. Home monitoring of your own sugar or glucose levels will enable you to give accurate information to your physician. Homeopathic care seeks to complement the team of health helpers you've probably assembled. As the next patient's story reveals, homeopaths aid you in managing your mind and body for overall health while addressing your particular susceptibility to blood sugar issues.

Diabetes (Presented by Savitri Clarke)

Ron walks into my office with a rather rigid gait. He seems quite anxious. He has recently been diagnosed with diabetes. He does not need insulin yet and would like to avoid that if at all possible. He used to be an "ice cream addict," but has had to stop. He also has stomach problems, which he describes as pain in the left side of his abdomen that is very sore to touch. He wakes at 4 A.M. with a growling stomach. "I feel like a truck ran over me, really sick, then it starts with gas gurgling, like bubbles bursting. It gets me out of bed and I feel that I have to have a bowel movement but it doesn't relieve. It is hard to get back to sleep because of the pain." He gets anxious with the pains and feels anxious just talking about it now.

Ron has been sober for 20 years. He worries about his health and thinks about it a lot. He can have trouble breathing when he is anxious. The diagnosis of diabetes was "devastating" to him. His body has become more and more stiff with arthritis. He is an amateur musician and playing music always makes him feel better. Exercise also helps.

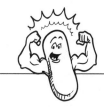

Potent Pellets

People with Type II (DM) are less able to perceive the sweet tastes in foods, making it more difficult to recognize sugary substances. They often have difficulty losing the weight that would help their overall condition.

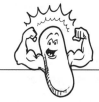

Potent Pellets

Researchers of a 16-year study announced that those who lost 8 to 15 pounds had a 33 percent reduction in risk of Type II (DM), while losing more weight decreased the risk by 51 percent.

There is a great deal of degenerative disease and early death in Ron's family which worries him. He describes himself as "always tense and jittery." His childhood was very difficult with both parents dying young. He was raised by an alcoholic uncle. He believes in following the rules and is upset if he thinks he hasn't. As Ron talks to me about his life, his work history, and his marriage I become aware that he has always wanted to feel important and has tried hard but has never really succeeded. His childhood was one of constant tension which is now quite evident in Ron's body which is always cramping up on him. I gave him Cuprum Metallicum.

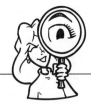

Curious Clues

The sensation of bubbles forming and bursting in the abdomen was an unusual symptom and led to the remedy Cuprum, homeopathic copper. Cuprum also has the following symptoms:

➤ Anxiety with difficult respiration

➤ Anxiety from the pain

➤ Cramping and tensions anywhere in the body

➤ Desire to follow rules and regulations

➤ Better from physical exertion

➤ Better from music

Ron returned after six weeks to report that, "The pain in my left side is 95 percent better and the gurgling is also 95 percent better, which is amazing to me!" He is happy to be getting some rest. His blood sugar has been lower and more stable. He exclaimed, "It is incredible. I feel like a human being again! I used to wake up and say I don't care if I wake up another day." Over the next two years Ron's digestive problem totally resolved and his blood sugar reduced and stayed within normal limits. He found himself worrying less and more able to relax and enjoy himself.

Mild Traumatic Brain Injury (MTBI)

How would it feel to check and recheck yourself at every turn, because you can't re- member what you've done. What about struggling with headaches, fatigue, sleep problems, dizziness, loss of sex drive, seizures, irritability, depression, or sudden ex- plosive temper since an automobile accident almost three months ago. That's what over two million Americans with mild traumatic brain injury (MTBI) can experience on a daily basis, yet only 22 percent receive hospital or medical attention. According to Dr. Diane Stoler, author of *Coping with Mild Traumatic Brain Injury*, of the more than 325,000 who receive a MTBI each year, thousands more go undiagnosed, be- cause no medical treatment is sought, despite troubling persistent after-effects of a head injury (Stoler, 1998).

There are two types of traumatic brain injuries (Stoler, 1998):

➤ **Open-head injury:** The skull is penetrated, and a specific area of the brain is damaged by the external force that causes the brain to swell.

➤ **Closed-head injury:** The skull is not penetrated, and brain damage occurs as a result of external force that causes the brain to move and slam into the skull.

Whenever your head is involved in a violent sudden motion, your soft floating brain gets smashed against the skull's uneven interior. The brain's threadlike nerve cells are stretched, strained, or torn. While the damage is microscopic, the results can be catastrophic.

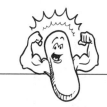

Potent Pellets

The causes of traumatic brain injury include automobile accidents: 50 percent; falls: 21 percent; violence, including physical abuse: 12 percent; sports and recreation: 10 percent (Stoler, 1998).

Mild traumatic brain injury (MTBI) is defined by a brief loss of consciousness and memory, lasting no longer than 60 minutes. Some people are fortunate by experiencing little or no symptoms after a week or two; however, 60 percent of people with MTBI still suffer with neurological problems three months after the injury.

Proper diagnosis seems to be one of the biggest challenges with finding qualified, experienced providers who recognize the symptoms and may order tests such as quantitative electroencephalogram (EEG) to look at nerve fibers, magnetic resonance imaging (MRI), or computed tomography (CT) scan for a better look at the brain. Conventional medical treatment includes prescribing drugs and therapy for the condition that the tests reveal, but not having a standard pharmacological approach.

Homeopathy has been the subject of a study written in the *Journal of Head Trauma and Rehabilitation*. The study suggests that homeopathy may have a role in treating persistent MTBI with test results showing significant improvement versus the control group. The patient's story gives a glimpse into what I believe is a good integration of homeopathy into a comprehensive medical team.

MTBI

"In one second, my whole life changed. One moment I was awake and alert, the next I was involved in a head-on automobile accident. Days later, my doctors diagnosed me as having suffered a mild traumatic brain injury," recalled Dina, who came to me for help with the healing process from the brain injury she received almost one year ago.

"Since I looked and felt fine, save for minor cuts and bruises, all I wanted to know was when could I return to work. I felt alone, none of my doctors fully explained my problems, told me what to expect, or explained how to cope."

249

Dina's physical symptoms were extensive. She experienced right-sided headaches, a numb triangle area on her right cheek, difficulty in speaking, loss of coordination, especially the use of her right hand, debilitating fatigue, difficulty in thinking and concentrating, with chronic muscle spasms and weakness of her neck, upper back, and shoulders.

She explained that she had taken numerous medications but had to get off them because of the side effects. She described herself as "hypersensitive to medications." She had been a diligent goal setter, ambitious in her professional career, and now stated she felt exhausted and "brain dead." She missed the life she had and would cry easily. She was very disappointed that her family was not more supportive. "I looked so good. I had to remind people that I'm still injured." She felt guilty if she couldn't do everything and felt like her family blamed her for not doing her part. She likes to be efficient but couldn't do it anymore. "I can only absorb so much before I can't handle it emotionally. I'm really burned out, stuck; what the hell am I doing wrong?"

Dina was very talkative, but I noticed she would stop talking if I was not making eye contact with her. When I jotted down notes or entered data on my laptop, she would pause until we looked at each other again. Her goals were to be a national speaker. She was outgoing and entertaining, but I had the feeling that she needed to be in absolute control of our sessions. She would direct me to topics that she wanted to discuss and away from others, dismissing them as unimportant. I gave her Bungaris.

How I felt being with Dina and her subtle manipulation and eye contact, combined with the strong right-sided physical paralysis and the stuck emotional state that she was experiencing, led me to Bungaris, a snake-derived homeopathic remedy.

Most people who would benefit from this remedy are also hypersensitive to medications, demand care taking, and are disappointed and angered not to get it. They can be very talkative and slanderous with their comments and have a desire to be the center of attention. A common snake trait is to magnetize you with their eyes, so eye contact is very important to them.

"I was better able to handle the horrible comments by my sons," Dina reported on her six-week follow-up. Muscle pain was better. She is still busy and tired but coping better. Concentration is better, and her speech is slurred only when she's tired. Over the next year and a half her symptoms gradually improved. She evolved emotionally, changing her life as she wished without being held back. Today she is an author and national speaker.

Cancer: The Balancing Act

Patients share with me the fine line they walk with undergoing the most physically and emotionally challenging period of their lives during the diagnosis and treatment of cancer. Their worlds are weighted by caring family and friends, new techniques, and hope on one side while their symptoms of doubt, fear, and uncertainty of treatment tugs on the other. Balancing becomes a full-time job.

Our bodies are amazing in the way trillions of cells are made and distributed through-out a complex network of systems. Normal cells grow, reproduce, and die in response to internal and external signals from our body. When normal cells mutate or change into cancer cells, then the problem begins.

Cancer is the abnormal growth, reproduction, and spread of body cells. These cells do not obey the normal signals of the body that control other cells and behave inde-pendently instead of working in harmony with your system. Sometimes cancer cells reproduce and form a lump or tumor. If the tumor is self-contained and doesn't spread, it's called benign and is usually surgically removed. If tumor cells grow, di-vide, and damage the normal cells around them and invade other tissue or travel through your bloodstream, it's called malignant or cancerous. Metastasis refers to a malignant tumor's cells that enter the bloodstream. The danger comes from the spread of these cancer cells to other tissues in your body where new tumors can grow.

As tumors grow and multiply, they rob your normal healthy cells of nutrients, caus-ing disruption in your body's ability to function. Deteriorating health or death usu-ally results. No one knows exactly why some cells become cancerous. Certain exposures or behaviors have been linked to cancer. It's common knowledge these days that exposure to cigarette smoke puts you at a significantly higher risk of lung cancer. A diet that is high in fat and low in fiber is associated with increased risk of colorectal cancer and is a factor in breast and prostate cancer, too.

Defining Your Cancer

Each cancer diagnosis is defined by four areas that let your health provider know where the tumor is and the progress it's made in your body:

➤ Site: The place where the cancer occurs (lung, skin, or breast)

➤ Stage: How much has the tumor grown or spread

Stage 1: Contained to original site

Stage 2: Spread to nearby lymph nodes or tissues

Stage 3: Spread to other tissues in your body

Stage 4: Cancer has begun in a large amount of tissue

A thorough treatment program involves a combi-nation of therapies to rid your body of disease, re-lieve pain, and keep you healthy. Conventional therapies include surgery, radiation therapy, chemotherapy, and hormone therapy. I encourage

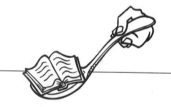

Dose of Info

Types of cancer include ...

➤ **Carcinoma:** Originates in the skin and lining of or-gans and glands.

➤ **Leukemia:** Cancer of blood-forming tissues.

➤ **Sarcoma:** Begins in connective tissue, bone, and cartilage.

➤ **Lymphoma:** Affects the lymphatic or immune system.

patients to find out about their condition, treatment options, and the possible side effects from undergoing the process.

I ask patients to inform their oncologist of their use of homeopathy and make myself available to answer any questions or concerns. Homeopathic treatment seeks to complement conventional care and not replace it. Strengthening your immune system, reducing potential side effects, and improving your overall health benefits are all concerned. The next patient's story will reflect the help that is available with homeopathic care.

Postcancer Support (Presented by Savitri Clarke)

Elaine is a 43-year-old woman who would like help with the after-effects of treatment for Non-Hodgkins Lymphoma. Two and a half years ago she had a gland on her neck swell to the size of an egg. At first she thought it was just a virus because she takes care of little children and they had all been sick. But the biopsy came back positive and Elaine received six rounds of chemotherapy over the next six months. "It was such a shock. There is no cancer in my family. I thought I did everything right. It was devastating. The worst thing was my children. My husband was a great support."

Elaine had a history of underactive thyroid. She took medicine for several years for symptoms of constipation, dry skin, bad yeast infections, and a very heavy menstrual period. She is always cold. In addition, Elaine gets migraine headaches, which are allergy related. They started when she was home with four young children. "I loved being home with my children. My husband worked long hours. I have always been a caretaker. My kids are older now so I do day care."

Elaine is very sensitive. "I can't read bad stories, it is too upsetting." Her parents were overprotective and strict. Her father had a heart attack when she was seven years old. "I know I worried about him. I worry a lot, about everyone." Elaine has prophetic dreams and feelings that she never tells anyone. "They would think I was crazy." As a child she was concerned how others would perceive her and she still is. "I was a perfectionist child. Behaved well, not a risk taker."

After the chemotherapy Elaine stopped getting her periods. Now she gets them sporadically. She is always constipated and has a bowel movement only once a week. She has a tremendous amount of bloating and loud, smelly gas. Elaine spends a lot of time taking care of others. It is important to her that everyone be protected and safe. She needs the support of her family and her husband. The remedy she needed was Calcaria Carbonica, or homeopathic calcium carbonate.

When Elaine returned six weeks later she described the changes she noticed. "I felt wonderful after I left here. The constipation is much better. I sleep better. I lost five pounds. Even my husband said I was doing great! I am not so tired and sluggish when I wake up. The funny thing is I never liked cats before. I guess I was always a little bit afraid of them. But now I love them! I feel so good, like I was before I was sick. And my period has come back two months in a row. I am moving more, walking more, and feeling good."

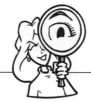

Curious Clues

Calcaria Carbonica comes from the oyster shell, which has a soft sensitive inside with a strong protective exterior. The remedy covered these symptoms:

➤ Fear of her condition being observed

➤ Constipation, inactivity of the rectum

➤ Always cold

➤ Heavy menstrual periods

➤ Horrible stories affect her profoundly

➤ Full of cares and worries

➤ Clairvoyance

➤ Delusion that she will become insane

Elaine continued to get stronger over the next six months with occasional doses of her remedy. Now that the effects of the cancer treatment are behind her, she feels happier and is enjoying her life like she used to with much less worrying.

The Facts on Fatigue

"The Syndromes of Uncertain Origin" is the heading under which you'll find chronic fatigue syndrome listed in the *Merck Manual,* a standard reference text for medical information (1999). The condition has become well known in this country, but the cause has not. Some experts believe this syndrome is linked to infection with the Epstein-Barr virus (EBV), which is the cause of mononucleosis. This is still controversial because it's never been satisfactorily proven. As in many syndromes, people suffer greatly from a variety of symptoms for which no specific reason can be found. People with chronic fatigue may have anemia, hypoglycemia, sleep problems, toxic exposures, emotional problems, hypothyroidism, and fungal infections such as *Candida albicans*. All have been thought to cause or contribute to the declining immune system found in this challenging condition.

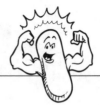

Potent Pellets

According to the *Merck Manual*, in addition to severe fatigue, chronic fatigue syndrome is diagnosed by experiencing at least four of these symptoms for over six months:

➤ Impaired short-term memory loss that interferes with work and social activities

➤ Sore throat

➤ Tender lymph nodes in neck or armpit

➤ Muscle pain

➤ Multijoint pain without swelling or tenderness

➤ Headaches, new pattern or severity

➤ Unrefreshing sleep

➤ More than 24 hours of fatigue following exertion

The symptom that usually gets your attention is the severe fatigue that wears you down. It is persistent and reoccurring, is not due to too much work, and is not relieved by rest. Women are three times more likely to have chronic fatigue syndrome, which mostly affects young adults between the ages of 20 and 40. The tragedy is that the symptoms are often debilitating, dramatically changing a person's lifestyle.

Treatment is often individualized because of the lack of identifiable cause. Conventional medical treatment uses antidepressants frequently, while many other agents are either inconclusive or disappointing in clinical trials. Homeopathy is perfectly suited to customize a well-chosen remedy around your individual experience of chronic fatigue. Building up your immune system and aiding your body in achieving balance of body, mind, and spirit are the goals of homeopathic care. My next patient's story will give you some insights to the process of homeopathic healing in chronic fatigue.

CFIDS (*Chronic Fatigue Immune Deficiency Syndrome*)

"Janet comes home from school and goes straight to bed exhausted," said Janet's mother, Evelyn. Janet was 17 years of age, a junior in high school who had been diagnosed with chronic fatigue syndrome after she began to miss many school days. She was so tired she either couldn't get out of bed, or fell asleep in class. They had tried several prescription medicines, only to see Janet's depression and fatigue change the girl they had known. Her digestion was normal, but she was just not hungry. I observed she frequently yawned during our interview. She complained of two or three days of PMS with a decrease in symptoms after the start of her menses. She had asthma and used a prescription inhaler with sinus congestion, facial pain, and headaches. She has been forgetful and concentration is increasingly difficult.

Before these symptoms began two years ago, she was lively, active in school and church. Her parents have taken away her driving privileges, because she has been experiencing suicidal thoughts. "I daydream about driving my car off the road and flipping it over," Janet says. Her parents have been with her on a 24-hour watch. "She cries at just about everything; she's sad and angry all the time," her mother says. "I don't like people in general. I want to hurt all the children that pick on me or my sisters." She began to slander many of the people in her life that she perceived as a threat. "I'm more aggressive than they are," she would say with a smile.

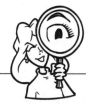

Curious Clues

Janet was coiled, inhibited, depressed, and quiet when tired. When rested, she exhibited more of the common snake-like qualities of aggression, sarcasm, and passion about her looks and life. Other Lachesis symptoms that confirmed the remedy for me included ...

➤ Overwhelming fatigue.

➤ Suicidal thoughts.

➤ Asthma.

➤ Premenstrual syndrome.

➤ Depression.

➤ Jealousy, envy.

Despite her overwhelming fatigue, Janet's looks were important. She would wear lots of jewelry and makeup, wished she had better clothes, and would say unkind remarks about other girls who had more money and better clothes. I gave Janet Lachesis, the diluted derivative of the bushmaster snake.

Janet returned for her six-week follow-up saying that she had felt generally better. "I have more energy to do the things I want to do." Suicidal thoughts and fantasies had steadily decreased as her depression slowly lifted. She was still very sensitive, angry mostly before her menses. She still experienced painful periods, but was less agitated. Her asthma also had improved.

Over the next few months, Janet was able to get off all her medications. She was still being seen by her physician and psychologist on a regular basis. Her moods became more level, even before her menstrual cycle, which also became less painful. Her asthma was not an issue, and she had not used her inhaler for a month. "I feel good," she said; she was socializing more, less critical and slanderous of others. She was going to school regularly and began volunteering at school and work.

As the practitioner, I want to be clear that since chronic fatigue is not clearly understood and reoccurrences can happen, I can't say that Janet is cured. She's felt good for more than three years now, is in college, and doing well. Homeopathic medicines have been used in many of the cases you've just read as a safe therapeutic option with all the other conventional medical practitioners on board, all working for the good of the patient.

The Least You Need to Know

➤ Homeopathy may be an excellent individualized therapeutic option for today's myriad of mysterious conditions.

➤ More than 5.5 million Americans are being treated for diabetes, with possibly another 5 million who don't even know they are diabetic.

➤ Automobile accidents account for about 50 percent of all traumatic brain injuries.

➤ Homeopathic care for cancer seeks to complement conventional care, not replace it.

➤ Chronic fatigue immune deficiency syndrome (CFIDS) is not well understood and can reoccur with periods of stress; homeopathy is used to help patients bolster their immune system and balance their lives.

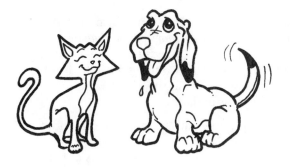

Veterinary Homeopathy

We smother our faithful companions with care and appreciation for their constant cuddling and love. Some of the most hilarious and heartfelt moments of our lives include our precious pets. When they are ill, we do our very best to find effective comprehensive care. You may want to look in your neighborhood for a homeopathic veterinarian to add to your team. The same complete healing system you've been reading about is available for your pets.

By taking careful notes of your pet's behavior before and after homeopathic medicine, good communication can exist with your homeopathic vet. While many of the mental and emotional symptoms would only be conjecture on our parts, you've spent a lot of time with your companion and can pass these insights on to your homeopathic vet.

This chapter will cover some of the homeopathic vet basics so that you can examine the issues and the benefits of including homeopathy as part of a comprehensive care plan for your loving companion.

Working with a Homeopathic Vet

You know the worrisome signs that signal a visit to your vet may be necessary. Don Hamilton, D.V.M., has written a comprehensive book, *Homeopathic Care for Cats and Dogs* (Hamilton, 1999). He outlines symptoms such as refusal to eat for a couple of days, breathing difficulties, frequent vomiting (one or two times a day if chronic, more if acute), persistent diarrhea, or weakness and listlessness lasting more than a day as reasons to seek assistance from your veterinarian.

The communication you establish with your homeopathic vet is essential for effective care. Using a notebook is a great way to record the physical symptoms and any behavioral changes. Also note what else is going on, such as the emotions of your family, time of day or week symptoms occur, food changes, weather circumstances, or under what circumstance things seem to get better or worse.

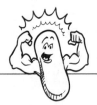

Potent Pellets

Homeopathic remedies are tested on people, not animals. Groups of volunteers under supervision take safe doses of diluted substances until they produce symptoms. These symptoms of a proving are carefully recorded and aid homeopaths in their understanding of how to effectively use these safe, nontoxic medicines.

Lady the Boxer Dog (Presented by Karen Komisar, D.V.M.)

Lady is a five-year old, female, spayed Boxer dog. She first was brought to my office with a history of dry flaky skin with a poor coat, black, cystic skin lumps, shortness of breath diagnosed as asthma, vomiting after drinking water, increased frequency of urination and cystitis (bladder inflammation), separation anxiety, colitis and a harsh barking cough called kennel cough. This would be named bronchitis if the patient were a person.

An interview with her guardian elicited the following information. Lady was a friendly dog, good with children, with a tendency to be overactive. She was slightly fearful around strangers and submissive around other dogs. She dislikes cold and will allow her guardian to cover her with a blanket. The guardian also felt that Lady was weak in the hind end although she was less than five years old. They also noted that Lady had a ravenous appetite. The current concern of the guardians centered on her diagnosis of inflammatory bowel disease. The symptoms of this included flatus, rumbling of the abdomen, and frequent vomiting of undigested food several hours after eating. At the time of the intake Lady had just completed a course of prednisone to control her asthma and bowel problem.

Conventional practitioners would view each of Lady's problems independently and treat them separately. As a homeopath, I reviewed the entire case and saw a consistent thread of inflammation throughout, and used this as a key to prescribing.

I started this case by prescribing Calcaria Carbonica. At the end of two weeks, Lady was vomiting less frequently and her wheezing had decreased. She had developed a rash between the pads of her feet, which I learned was an old symptom that had been treated with steroids in the past. An old symptom returning confirmed we were on the right track. We continued with the remedy and over the next six months saw her problems resolve.

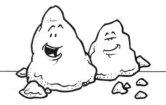

Natural Nuggets

Pet remedies are given orally like other medications or can be mixed with a small amount of milk. The pet then drinks the milk.

In February 1998, Lady became more fearful and experienced an increase in her flatulence. I prescribed Argentum Nitricum given one time. A week after the Argentum Nitricum was given, Lady vomited blood and mucus, which occurred only one time. By the middle of March, Lady's mental symptoms had improved but she was again vomiting more frequently. I changed her remedy to Phosphorus LM. The remedy change was due to the symptom change. Remedies are administered for the state the animal is in. As this dog's vital force shifted, her remedy needed to shift too. LM potencies are an administrative form of homeopathic remedies used when the vital force is weak or the risk of aggravation of symptoms is present.

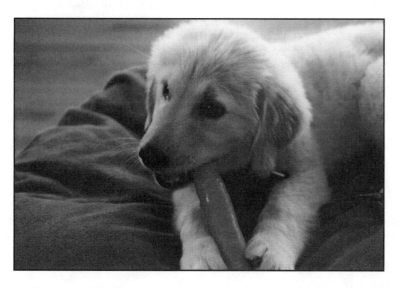

Daisy Crawford, a golden retriever puppy, is happy chewing on the recommended fresh vegetables. She is a patient of Dr. Komisar's, using homeopathics for her continuing health.

On evaluation in the office in late March, Lady had a pimple-like skin eruption on her chest, her vomiting was decreased, and she had a grade II heart murmur present when I listened to her internal organs with a stethoscope. She was evaluated by a cardiologist for signs of cardiomyopathy (common in this breed) and was found to have no evidence of organic heart disease. We continued with the Phosphorus LM.

In June 1998, the skin lesion was still present. Lady no longer vomited food, but occasionally vomited bile and had gas. Her fear symptoms were improved and she still liked to be warm. Her remedy was changed to Arsenicum Album administered one time.

At her one-month follow-up, the vomiting was decreased further and the skin lesion had resolved. Two weeks later, the guardians called to say there was a return of symptoms. She was given Arsenicum Album. Lady received Arsenicum Album in increasing potency each time her symptoms recurred over an eight-month period. At that time Lady received her rabies vaccination. After her rabies vaccination, Lady developed an increase in the frequency of gas and vomiting; she also became very attached and clingy with her owner. I prescribed Pulsitilla. Lady did very well for five months.

Three years after beginning treatment homeopathically, Lady has a beautiful coat, no respiratory symptoms. She is friendly and outgoing, and has a normal appetite. Her guardians are thrilled with her progress.

Diet: Your Nutrition Mission

I remember my dog Butch putting on airs of entitlement when our dinner was served. He did not beg; he sat waiting until he was served. At the time we were embarrassed we were feeding our dog from the table, but now I learn we may have been contributing in a positive way to his health. According to Dr. Don Hamilton, the best parameter for evaluation of a diet is the reaction by your companion. He states that normal response to dietary changes takes a good six months to notice discernable progress, with a year or two to view the maximum improvement with very ill animals. Animals in the wild eat raw foods such as meats and vegetables. Fresh-cooked meats, grains, vegetables, and supplements may also work well to create a balanced diet. Use organic foods whenever possible, especially with organ meats like liver and kidneys. Nonorganic organ meats expose your animal to high amounts of harmful substances like pesticides, antibiotics, and steroids.

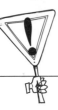

Caution Keeper

Beware of commercial pet food lists of hideous ingredients: rotten meats and rancid oils, diseased animal parts, cats and dogs killed at shelters, some still wearing their flea collars that become part of the food, as do the drugs that killed them (Hamilton, 1999).

Just as in humans, you can't expect your pet to have great health from poor foods and nutrition. When switching to a better diet, make the individual changes gradually and keep checking your progress with the one who counts: your faithful companion!

Casey, an Australian shepherd puppy, shares her story of health and healing the homeopathic way.

Casey the Australian Shepherd Puppy (Presented by Karen Komisar, D.V.M.)

Casey is a blue merle Australian shepherd puppy. She had a very rocky start in life. A child in the Midwest found her and a litter mate as strays. They were rescued and were kept in a shelter until adopted. At the time of adoption, the dogs were estimated to be 14 weeks old.

Within a few days of her first vaccination, Casey developed diarrhea. She was diagnosed with an intestinal parasite and treated with antibiotics. Within one week of finishing her antibiotic therapy, Casey developed a cough that progressed to pneumonia. Her pneumonia was severe and required hospitalization. She was treated with a dual course of antibiotics. Upon recovering from her pneumonia, Casey developed a neurologic condition in her left hind leg. She was treated with anti-inflammatory drugs and vaccinated again. Two weeks later, the pain in the hind leg worsened and she was treated with anti-inflammatory medication. As soon as she was weaned off her medication, Casey underwent a hysterectomy.

Casey had a variety of infectious and neurological problems when we met. The owner was willing to acknowledge that Casey's symptoms had indeed subsided; however, she was left with a juvenile animal that acted more like an elderly dog. Casey's poor appetite and lack of energy from a traditional respect did not require treatment since her symptoms had resolved. Casey's guardian wanted something more for her and so sought out homeopathic treatment.

The chief complaint was lack of energy and poor appetite. I would have expected a six-month old dog to be a rambunctious puppy, curious and active in new surroundings. Instead the dog that I saw was subdued, quiet and responsive, but with little of the attitude I would have expected. Other than lethargy and lack of appetite, there were few other symptoms apparent. Casey had no temperature preferences, was eating a good diet, and got along well with the other animals and people in her life. Based upon her history and presenting signs, I sent Casey home with Sulphur to be given daily for one week. The guardian was to report at the end of the week. When the guardian called, she was delighted. Casey was eating well and was more active than she had ever been. It has been four months since her remedy and she continues to do well.

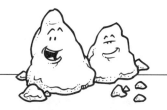

Natural Nuggets

When farm animals are treated solely with natural homeopathic medicines, there is no chemical residue in the meat, eggs, or dairy products.

Source: Homeopathy Today, February 1997

Vaccination: Hesitation?

Vaccinations are controversial in human health care, so it's no surprise that a growing number of veterinarians, not just homeopaths, are questioning the value and weighing the risks of this treatment. A vaccine is a suspended live or dead microorganism administered into the body for prevention, amelioration, or treatment of infectious diseases. Historically vaccinations have stopped epidemics of infectious diseases, such as rabies in domestic animals in the 1950s, feline rhinotracheitis epidemic in the late 1960s, and the canine parvovirus epidemic in the 1970s.

The controversy continues with veterinarians looking at the incidence of harmful side effects and examining the necessity of such legal and medical standards as boosters. Dr. Don Hamilton states in his book that "yearly vaccination is unscientific." He goes on to say that "old-dog encephalitis," a form of canine distemper, was vaccinated against and thought to have a lapse in immunity with time. So a repetition of vaccination was needed. "This theory," he states, "was never proven, but the practice of 'boosters' continued despite the questionable results and potential problems that this may create for your companion."

Vaccination may prevent specific diseases in the short term, but the usefulness as a prevention method is less certain, according to Dr. Don Hamilton. I suggest educating yourself about this important issue.

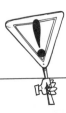

Caution Keeper

European Union scientists are recommending immediate cuts in the use of antibiotics and other microbial products. Growing bacterial resistance to antibiotics has led to increasing difficulties with treating diseases such as pneumonia, tuberculosis, and salmonella. The European Council has already decided to have four antibiotics used as growth promoters on July 1, 1999.

Homeopathic Vets Across the Pond

Since homeopathy began in Europe and has continued to be integrated in these countries in some form, we can expect to find more uses in treating animals. The European Council for Classical Homeopathy (ECCH) recently conducted a survey of 15 countries including the United Kingdom, Germany, France, Greece, Switzerland, and Portugal, and found that homeopathic vets were treating animals in all countries.

In some countries, just as state by state in the United States, veterinarians are the only ones who can legally practice homeopathy on animals. Education varies from basic seminars to one- to two-year courses in comprehensive theory and homeopathic prescribing.

The European Union has been busy organizing homeopathic regulations. In 1992, two directives dealt with homeopathic accessibility, safety, information for users, preparation, and supervision of the medicines. In the United States, the Academy of Veterinary Homeopathy

(704-535-6688) and the American Holistic Veterinary Medical Association (410-569-0795) support practitioners and maintain a list of veterinarians who have been certified by these organizations.

Sugar is a female beagle dog whose story will illustrate the life quality benefits that homeopathy can offer you and your companion.

Sugar the Female Beagle Dog (Presented by Karen Komisar, D.V.M.)

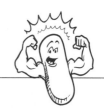

Sugar's diagnosis was idiopathic epilepsy. Epilepsy is the occurrence of random electrical discharges in the brain resulting in seizure activity. There are many causes of epilepsy, which must be ruled out before beginning therapy. Sugar's epilepsy was diagnosed as idiopathic, meaning no known organic cause. The treatment protocol that had been recommended to her guardians included barbiturates and potassium bromide. Traditional treatment for epilepsy is lifelong therapy once it has begun. Sugar is a four-year-old, spayed female beagle dog. She was adopted from an animal shelter and had been with her new family about six months when she started to have epileptic seizures. Her guardians were reluctant to start her on lifelong drug therapy and so came to me for a homeopathic alternative.

Potent Pellets

A Swedish survey showed that 14 percent of milk-producing farmers are regularly using homeopathy to treat their animals. The main reason stated by the farmers was the risk of bacterial resistance when using antibiotics.

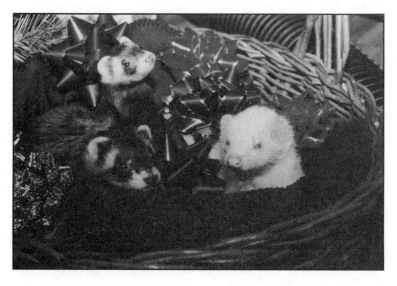

Janet, Pickles, and Peter (left to right) are a basket of ferret-family fun, cared for by good nutrition, homeopathics, and heartfelt love.

Sugar was a shy dog. She was fearful of strange noises, strange places, and men. Her coat was dry and flaky. Her ears were chronically inflamed and had yeast present. She also needed to urinate frequently. At home she is a "couch potato." Based upon her presentation I prescribed Silicea.

After a three-month period of no seizures, I discovered Sugar had a rectal polyp. I gave her a dose of Thuja, and two weeks later the polyp fell off. She has continued to do well since that time.

The search for optimal health for your companion is of the highest priority in homeopathic care. These principles, as we've discussed with human well-being, focus on building immunity, promoting health, and creating a supportive lifestyle with diet and exercise. Veterinarian homeopathy frames health in the same way, instead of focusing on fighting a disease. I encourage you to contact a homeopathic vet near you and learn the options that await you and your loving companion.

The Least You Need to Know

➤ Keep a notepad to track your pet's progress in between visits.

➤ Homeopathic medicines are tested safely on humans, not animals.

➤ Organic raw or cooked foods are best for your pets' healthy diet.

➤ Check the ingredients of your commercial pet foods for rancid meats and diseased animals.

➤ Have a discussion with your vet about the necessity of vaccinations for your companion.

➤ The European Union has recommended cutting back on antibiotics due to growing bacterial resistance to antibiotics used to treat pneumonia, tuberculosis, and salmonella.

Part 5

Integration and Participation

Homeopathy is not a spectator sport. It's time to suit up and get into the game. We'll take a scouting trip together so that you will know what to expect on your follow-up appointment and how important giving 110 percent really is to the therapeutic team.

Any sand traps on this course? You bet! I'll guide you through the obstacles of generics, conventional medicine, and the limits of homeopathy while giving you pointers on using all the medical tools in your bag to help you and your family.

I'll show you how to get your doctor into the huddle. With help and guidance, the rest is up to you. The good news is that you're the best one for the job. I'll share some secrets from my playbook, so being your own head coach is not a headache, but fun. I'll look for you at the goal line. Go get 'em, tiger!

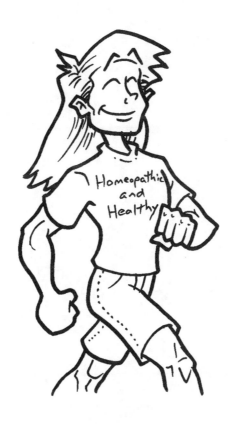

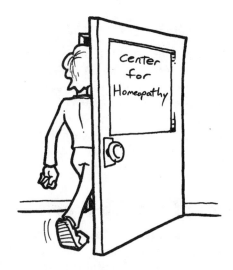

Chapter 23

Your Return Visit

> ## In This Chapter
>
> ➤ Learn what's important to tell your homeopath during your follow-up visit
>
> ➤ Is your remedy working? Find out how to know for sure
>
> ➤ Discover the choices your practitioner makes for your second homeopathic prescription
>
> ➤ Treating yourself with homeopathy? Read for some pointers ahead

In most cases, you've been interacting with the world for four to eight weeks after taking your homeopathic remedy. What's been going on and how can your homeopath tell if you're getting better? This chapter focuses on the follow-up visit to your homeopath. I hope you'll understand what's important to a homeopath and the process that's involved in measuring your success with the homeopathic remedy that you've been given.

I'll walk you step-by-step through the typical choices that your homeopath will face at the moment of truth. Are you thinking of treating yourself and your family with homeopathy? We'll discuss the pros and cons so your journey for health will get off on the right track. Sit back—the hard work is over. It's time to begin your own success story.

Your Follow-Up Visit: Reporting and Sorting

Your homeopath will use the same listening and observational skills that he or she used on your first visit to gauge the self-healing since you started taking the remedy. My patients often kid me about my open-ended questions, "How have you been this month? What's it been like for you?" or, "Anything else?" I am striving to be what Samuel Hahnemann refers to as "the unprejudiced observer," allowing space for your true self to emerge and say what's important to you. As homeopaths, we eventually decide if the remedy was a good match for you. Are the same individual characteristics still present or have they progressed in the direction to healing?

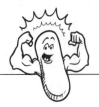

Potent Pellets

The unprejudiced observer, even the most sharp-witted one, perceives nothing in each single case of disease other than the alterations in the condition of the body and soul that are outwardly discernable through the senses. The unprejudiced observer ony perceives the deviations from the formerly healthy state of the now sick patient (O'Reilly, 1996).

The Truth Shall Set You Free

Homeopaths must choose a remedy based on what they observe. Sometimes a patient may hold back valuable information because he doesn't believe it to be important, or because of the discomfort he may experience telling a total stranger intimate details of his life. This is quite understandable. Sometimes it takes a couple of appointments to develop that trust. Once a homeopath has heard the patient's real concerns, the remedy choice becomes much clearer.

I had seen a man named Will for chronic allergies who always wanted to give me good news about his progress on a remedy. We have a great rapport, but I was finding remedies that only helped a little. Will did not want to tell me about his insecurities, how he had been victimized and abused throughout his life, because he didn't want me to think less of him. His conventional physicians had never asked him about it. Only after learning more about homeopathy did he say what was truly on his mind. I prescribed Silicae, and Will has been allergy-free since, plus his self-esteem has increased significantly and he is able to set appropriate boundaries.

Can a Remedy Make You Worse?

"You've got to get worse before you can get better" or "No pain, no gain" are both common sayings that mentally prepare us for what many call the healing crisis. I believe that more accurate prescribing by homeopaths combined with a larger selection of quality remedies and potencies have reduced the discomfort often associated with jump-starting your own healing energies.

Homeopathic aggravations are an increase in symptoms following the first dose of a remedy, which are usually temporary, lasting a few hours to a day. Some patients are very sensitive, and the remedies may temporarily overstimulate their systems. Often the person describes feeling better even though a symptom might be more strongly expressed. The key concept is that this does not last long, and they feel great or the same afterward. I've also had patients who had a flare-up of one of their symptoms, while everything else calmed down.

It reminds me of Alex, a nine-year-old boy who came in for treatment of eczema. After his first remedy, his mother panicked, because his eczema looked much worse despite Alex not being bothered by it. With patience and conversation, within about six weeks, not only the eczema but his allergies and many emotional concerns also went away. That was three years ago, and they've not returned.

Talk to your homeopath if you have any concerns about your symptoms getting worse.

Stopping Your Remedy from Working: Myth and Methods

There has been a significant amount of confusion regarding the methods of stopping or interfering with the homeopathic process. Patients are often panicked at having accepted the after-dinner mint or a stick of gum offered to them, thinking that might stop their remedy from working.

I consulted with several of my colleagues before writing this section. The consensus is that a well-chosen remedy will stimulate healing in your vital force and is not always affected by mint toothpaste or a cup of coffee. In Europe, where homeopathy has flourished for two centuries, they drink very strong coffee and still experience improvement from remedies. There are, however, individuals who are sensitive to certain substances like coffee and mints. In these cases, the remedies' progress could be interfered with or may themselves aggravate the patient's general or specific condition. For these people, avoiding substances like coffee and mint make sound sense. Careful evaluation by your homeopath can usually uncover the likelihood of this. Herbal products and conventional medications, especially steroids, can often cloud your body's reaction to a remedy or slow down your progress by suppressing symptoms; in my opinion, a good remedy keeps on going.

Is It Working? The Need for Speed

In an age of drive-through dry-cleaning, instant pudding, and one-hour photo processing, it is challenging to remind patients that our bodies can heal at slightly different rates. Drugs can mask symptoms often in a very short period of time, but if you stop taking the medications, you're often right back where you started. Homeopathy can also act with amazing speed, especially if the condition is acute or the remedy selected is a great match.

I remember a patient named Barry who came for a consultation for the chronic burning pain caused by shingles that had wrapped around his scalp and into his right eye. He was in almost unbearable pain. I gave him the homeopathic remedy I selected, put the bottle back in my cabinet, and before I sat down he thanked me because his pain had almost completely disappeared! It never returned during the following years, and he escorted the rest of his family in for treatment.

Ask yourself how you feel. Homeopathic healing spreads through the whole body and mind. Sound a little overwhelming to keep track of it all? Don't worry, that's why you have a trusted homeopath on your team.

Signs the Remedy Is Working Well

Taking stock of all your symptoms and judging progress is a team event. Check in with your homeopath who can help explain the process you're going through. Symptoms that show you're headed in the right direction of healing include …

➤ Stirring up of symptoms.

➤ Feeling better, then returning to original condition, then steady improvement.

➤ Superficial symptoms return, but you still feel good.

➤ Superficial symptoms come and go.

➤ Superficial symptoms get worse, yet you feel better.

➤ Short aggravation, then rapidly feeling better.

➤ Recovery without aggravation.

➤ Return of old symptoms while feeling generally good.

➤ Disappearance of superficial symptoms.

Signs the Remedy Is Not the Right One

Despite their best efforts, homeopaths do not always choose the best remedy the first time. Here are a few unwelcome symptoms that signal that a change may be in order:

➤ Very short period of feeling better

➤ Prolonged stirring up of superficial symptoms with extremely slow improvement

➤ Prolonged aggravation of superficial symptoms, with no improvement in overall health

➤ No change in symptoms

➤ Superficial symptoms are better, but you feel generally worse

➤ Appearance of new symptoms that you've never had before

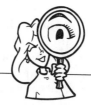

Curious Clues

Diane and Stan both had eczema. Diane was seven years old with learning and behavior challenges. Stan was 50 with arthritis and a high-powered job. After giving them both homeopathic remedies, Diane's eczema cleared up quickly, while her developmental delays improved significantly over the next year. Stan's arthritis dramatically improved so that he could function at work, play golf, and bowl again. His eczema took more than one year to finally go away. The key is they both had steady improvement in their specific complaints as well as overall health. The order was different, the results the same: freedom.

Can I Treat Myself with Homeopathy?

Homeopathy enjoys a long, safe history over the past two centuries with many families throughout the world having been shown by their relatives or family physician how to work with remedies. Europe and India have deeply integrated homeopathic traditions in their cultures that foster education and understanding about the process of healing.

As you've read in Chapter 2, "The Evolution of Homeopathy," and Appendix D, "A Brief History of Homeopathy," homeopathy in the United States has only flourished in the past few decades after a tragic decline. During that time, educational opportunities for families and professionals were extremely limited. Now we have abundant resources of books, burgeoning homeopathic organizations, homeopathic study groups, and clinics to encourage the education to spread once again. While self-prescribing generally is safe, I would also ask, "Is it effective?"

I talk to patients about "The Pepto-Bismol Model." We've probably all seen Pepto-Bismol commercials on TV, in drugstores, and maybe even been given it as children by a well-intentioned parent. All these experiences educated us about the proper use of the product. If you didn't get well within a day or two, you'd make an appointment to see your

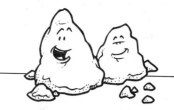

Natural Nuggets

Homeopathic training programs and study groups in your local area are great ways to learn responsible use of homeopathic medicines. One such organization is The National Center for Homeopathy, 801 N. Fairfax, #306, Alexandria, VA 22314, 707-548-7790, www.homeopathic.org.

health-care provider. If you didn't understand what was going on, you'd go straight to someone else you thought might help. This is how I view responsible use of homeopathic medicines. Do you have sufficient training to help? Great if you do. I prefer to refer my patients to specialists if their condition is beyond my understanding or experience. The twists and turns of a chronic condition, even when it improves, can sure test the skill and willpower of a homeopath.

Professional homeopaths have been learning during their entire career to help you have better health. Knowing your limits is an important sign of progress in understanding the process of healing.

The Second Prescription: Red, Yellow, or Green Light?

After your follow-up appointment, your homeopath will have some choices to discuss with you. Do you wait (red light), proceed with the same remedy at perhaps a stronger potency (yellow light), or move ahead to a new remedy all together (green light)?

We have to ask again, "Are you feeling better, and how are you better?" Having clear understanding of how a patient is progressing is essential to his continuing health. Let's review the possibilities of the second prescription.

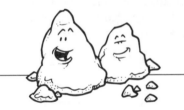

Natural Nuggets

You may administer a dozen remedies without them having any effect. Consider the first prescription the one that has affected changes, and subsequent to that the next prescription is the second (Kent, 1981).

The Toughest Pill to Swallow

This is often the most difficult prescription for a patient to get. We're all geared up to "do something" that fits our go-for-it, get-it-done society, and I suggest waiting as the best way to allow my patients' systems to continue to heal.

If you have been fortunate enough to have gotten a homeopathic remedy that has been helpful for you, waiting will give you and your homeopath the time to evaluate the needs of your body to keep the healing going. Remember that your magnificent body and mind continue to strive for healing perfection continuously without your homeopath's conscious permission or guidance.

Putting the Remedy to the Test

Your homeopath may decide to continue with the same remedy, perhaps modifying the strength and potency of the remedy or suggesting a change in frequency. Let's say you were using a 30c homeopathic remedy for a few days in a row. Your symptoms improved for a while and then returned to a stand-still. You may receive the same potency, or perhaps be given a higher strength (such as 200c) taken only once to activate your system that seemed to respond to the first prescription.

The rule of thumb here is to keep using a remedy that has proven to be helpful as long as you continue to improve. Careful attention must be used to have a clear understanding of the progress. Too many new remedies are chosen in haste when the old one was working just fine. Good communication and observational skills are needed to keep you on the right track.

New Remedy: Next!

You've waited and still had no change in your condition. You've tried different potencies without even the glimmer of an effect. This feeds your impatience, but it may be time for a new remedy; the old one seems to have missed the mark.

A patient may have been helped enough to reduce or get off all his conventional drugs, and both patient and practitioners are viewing a whole new set of symptoms and concerns. When such dramatic insight occurs that no longer matches the current remedy, a change is often called for. Also, if there has been no change and your condition continues to worsen, changing your homeopathic remedy becomes an option. I emphasize again that patience and good prescribing habits that you've just read about are essential to avoid snap judgments. Change in this case can be good for you!

Your follow-up visit is a great time to share your experiences and sensations with your homeopath. It is common to have new insights or realizations about yourself or your condition that were triggered by the remedy or the initial interview itself. Your homeopath is eager to listen. The first visit is so action-packed that a follow-up is often a better time to discuss the remedy choice and the questions you may have about the homeopathic process.

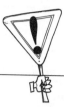

Caution Keeper

In *Lectures on Homeopathic Philosophy*, James T. Kent warns us to exercise patience and avoid rushing into giving a second prescription. "If the doctor administers a well-chosen remedy and repeats it too soon, he never gives the symptoms a chance to come back and call for a second prescription, but they come intermingled ... so a rational second prescription cannot be made" (Kent, 1979).

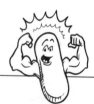

Potent Pellets

When the dose of a higher potency has been given and tested without effect, that is the only means you have of knowing that this remedy has done all the good it can for this patient and that a change is necessary (Kent, 1981).

The Least You Need to Know

➤ Homeopaths strive to be "unprejudiced observers" while listening to your experiences since the last visit.

➤ Sharing the truth during an office visit helps your homeopath know what is important to you.

➤ It takes a lot to stop a well-prescribed homeopathic remedy from working.

➤ Improving on the physical and emotional level are important signs of progress when using homeopathic medicines.

➤ Self-healing with homeopathy requires education and experience to ensure satisfactory results.

➤ Clear communication is essential when choosing to wait, repeat, or start a new remedy at your next appointment.

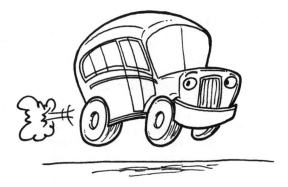

Chapter 24

Who's Driving Your Health Bus?

In This Chapter

➤ Discover the differences and similarities between conventional medicine and homeopathy

➤ Learn the limits of homeopathy

➤ Find out how your family tree may affect your health

➤ How to integrate homeopathy into your health-care team

Who chooses the direction of your health care, you or your health-care provider? Paul Schoonman, who works with me at our clinic as a chiropractic physician, uses this question to find out who's in charge. Are you sitting in the back of the bus, letting others drive your health and map out the road you'll travel, or are you at the wheel? There is a growing trend in health care where you sit at the wheel and have your practitioner and advisors counsel you during the journey. At times you may move them closer to you depending on your needs, while keeping your hands firmly on the wheel, alert to the choices and the turns up ahead. After all, you are the only one who'll be paying the toll.

In this chapter, we'll look at how homeopathy compares with conventional medicine. I hope you'll start getting ideas of how to use both to your advantage. We'll discuss the limitations and expectations of our dynamically diluted remedies, and I'll give you guidance about speaking with your physician about your health-care choices.

Homeopathy and Conventional Medicine: A Dissimilar Duo

Whether your practitioner adheres to the philosophies of *homeopathy* or conventional medicine, also known as *allopathy,* your practitioner's true intent is to help you the best way he or she knows how.

The philosophies of these medical models are what eventually collided at the turn of the last century, resulting in unnecessarily harsh dividing lines and an uncooperative spirit between them. Today both kinds of medicines are making strides toward finding integrated health solutions for the benefit of the patient.

Here are the basic philosophical differences between the homeopathic and allopathic view of health and healing. Finding a way to bridge these gaps is the challenge we now face.

Homeopathy vs. Allopathy

Homeopathy	Allopathy
Symptoms are seen as the body's best attempt to regain health	Symptoms are viewed as something wrong that must be fixed
Looks for the total picture and individual characteristics of illness	Look at the general symptoms of the illness
Similar general symptoms may require different medicines that are customized for the patient	Similar general symptoms are usually treated with the same medications
Treatment's aim is to restore complete health	Treatment is aimed at stopping or suppressing the general symptom
Complete restoration of health without the use of medications	Controls illnesses with regular use of medical drugs
Health means total freedom on physical, emotional, and mental levels	Health is the absence of disease

There are certainly sharp differences in the basic philosophies and practice of homeopathy and conventional allopathic medicine. *You* are the person in charge of your health, and finding the areas where each will perform well is *your* job. Look for more research and your own experience to help guide you and your family to safe and effective choices.

The Limits of Homeopathy

The healing help that most families ask for is during the course of their normal active lives. Few of us can check into a spa for a month and focus only on healing. We have to deal with the pressures of work and the stress of juggling family and professional commitments, while keeping enough health reserve to get up and do it all again tomorrow. Sound familiar? I ask my patients to think of a two-panned balancing scale, similar to the scales of justice on the statues. What are you putting on the healthful side and what is deposited on the unhealthful side? Do they balance? Sometimes I'm limited in my ability to help a patient who refuses to change detrimental health habits such as living next to a dump, poor diet, and lack of exercise. Homeopathy uses the spark from your own vital force to unite your body's healing powers. A stressful or unhealthy environment will hold back your chances of complete restoration of health.

Medications, especially steroids, may suppress symptoms, making it difficult or impossible for a homeopath to recognize the remedy that is most needed. During the time of homeopathy's creation, opium was used to mask pain; leeches, bleeding, and harsh purgatives were used to clean impurities from the body. These treatments often left the patient's system, or vital force, so weakened that homeopathy could not fully help. It's still true today. Severe illness, acute or chronic, coupled with a low vital force of the patient will still hinder the affect of homeopathy on your body. Remedies plus solid medical and nutritional management are needed to revive your health. Homeopathy can assist all along the way. As your health improves and your dependence on allopathic medications is minimized, homeopathy can play an increasingly vital role.

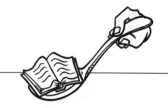

Dose of Info

The great divide in medical philosophy:

➤ **Allopathy (conventional medicine)**: The treatment of disease using medicines whose effects are different from those of the disease being treated. The medicines have no relationship to the symptoms of disease.

➤ **Homeopathy:** A system of therapeutics based on the administration of minute doses of substances that are capable of producing in healthy persons symptoms similar to those of the disease being treated.

Source: Dolan's Medical Dictionary

Genetic Influences: The Family Tree

The recent breakthroughs in human genetic research have much of the country buzzing about the power of the gene. During Samuel Hahnemann's time, science was in its infancy. He used his observational skills to conclude that some characteristics

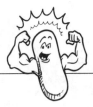

Potent Pellets

Do you like Parmesan cheese? The town, Parma, in Italy is known to make the best Parmesan cheese. A crucial ingredient for the great taste of their cheese is friendly bacteria that are present in the milk. Their secret? The cows have been treated homeopathically for the last 100 years to avoid using antibiotics that would also kill the healthy bacteria needed to make premium Parmesan cheese.

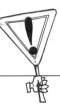

Caution Keeper

Samuel Hahnemann wrote: "As a result of the persistent repetition of unfitting medicines [allopathic] ... a new artificial chronic disease is added to the old natural disease, thus making the individual doubly diseased, much more diseased and more incurable, sometimes even entirely incurable" (O'Reilly, 1996).

and symptoms were passed on from parents to children, who also developed similar physical and emotional illnesses. Without the aid of technology, Hahnemann thought it was caused by an infection (like a virus) that would inhabit the organism and create similar susceptibility to certain diseases.

Homeopaths believe that the greatest good we can do for a patient is to help him lessen or eliminate the torments from his family tree. When I treat small children, their parents are usually very concerned when they see some of their childhood illnesses (such as eczema, asthma, allergies, or developmental delays) surface in their own child. They also watch in horror as their child displays similar issues of anger, worry, jealousy, and violence that they have had to deal with during their lives.

Homeopathy seeks to stop the cycle of susceptibility with well-chosen remedies that reflect the particular, unique, and characteristic symptoms. While challenging to test, I do see generations of chronic conditions that have not surfaced in the children whose parents have undergone homeopathic treatment for their own conditions. It's an added bonus to feeling good.

Adding Homeopathy to Your Team

Bringing in a homeopath is just like bringing in any other medical consultant. Most practitioners are happy to make contact with other medical providers to help foster a sense of open communication when treating you and your family. Remember that you are part of a growing trend in health care. Estimates of use of alternative medicines in this country range from 33 percent to over 45 percent with most people seeking help for chronic conditions. Unite your health-care providers to bring the best care possible for you and your family.

How to Talk with Your Doctor About Homeopathy

Amy was two years of age when she was brought in by her parents for treatment of chronic ear infections. Her pediatrician had prescribed five rounds of antibiotics, and Amy had been on a low-dose antibiotic for approximately one year. We began homeopathy with some nutritional changes and with her pediatrician fully informed, they stopped the antibiotics. Amy progressed well, as did her baby sister, mother, and later her father, who all underwent homeopathic care. Happy ending? Almost.

It turns out that they never talked to their pediatrician about homeopathy and their doctor still thinks they're all on antibiotics. When they started to bring it up, they got "a funny look" from their doctor and chose to keep silent rather than lose a pediatrician they might need later.

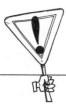

Caution Keeper

This is how Samuel Hahnemann explained his observations of chronic influences and how these chronic susceptibilities can be the starting point for many of our illnesses: "The greatest tormentors of our earthy existence, the tenders to countless diseases under which tormented humanity has been sighing for centuries and millennia" (O'Reilly, 1996).

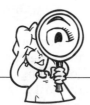

Curious Clues

Ten-year-old Shirley was accompanied by her mother and aunt on her first consultation for chronic sinusitis and asthma. Homeopathy had helped Shirley's mother and aunt, so they wanted her to feel well, too. I prescribed Chromium Metallicum for the general symptoms of thick, stringy, sticky yellow and green nasal discharge, and her particular signs of a controlling nature to avoid failure, criticism, and nervous anticipation. Within a month, her asthma was much improved, and she had a more relaxed personality. She did very well over the next six months. Today she does not complain of these symptoms. I hope that there will be a break in the family susceptibility so that her children will not have the same illnesses.

I believe that the best care comes from well-informed patients and practitioners. Here are a few tips to get the process going:

➤ Inform your medical doctor about seeing a homeopath.

➤ Discuss your reasons for seeking help with homeopathy.

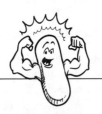

➤ Share with your doctor what you've learned about homeopathy and give him articles or Web site addresses that your homeopath recommends.

➤ Let your doctor know what you are taking (homeopathics, vitamins, herbs), and direct him to your practitioner to answer questions.

➤ Foster teamwork. Suggest that your doctor and homeopath connect to discuss your case.

➤ Reassure your doctor he's still part of your health-care team.

➤ Let him know how you feel about his reactions, positive or negative; keep the lines of communication open.

➤ Acknowledge openness and understanding.

This chapter has dealt with building bridges between two different philosophies for the good of your health, something that is often easier said than done! I believe the goal is worth pursuing if we are to achieve a medical system flexible enough to choose the best therapy—regardless of philosophy—available for optimal patient care and satisfaction.

Potent Pellets

According to a new study, the three principal reasons women don't talk to their medical doctors about alternative treatments are ...

➤ They feel the doctors aren't interested.

➤ Doctors have negative responses.

➤ Doctors don't have adequate information about alternative medicine or will have a bias against it.

Source: International Council on Women's Health Issues, January 27, 2000

The Least You Need to Know

➤ Homeopathy and allopathy (conventional medicine) have contrasting views on patient care and medical philosophy.

➤ An unhealthful lifestyle and suppressive medications limit the benefits from homeopathy.

➤ Homeopathic medical practices seek to lessen or eliminate the illnesses and susceptibilities that run in families.

➤ Communication and education with all your medical providers is the key to optimal coordinated health care.

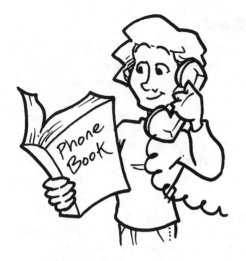

Chapter 25

Hunting for a Homeopath

In This Chapter

➤ Clues for finding your ideal homeopath

➤ Learn about homeopathic education

➤ Find out about state and federal laws regarding homeopathy

➤ Discover the role that women continue to play in this evolving medical art

➤ Confirmation on how follow-through still pays off

You're ready to take the next step in your journey by finding the best homeopath for you. This chapter delves into the practical issues of learning about the laws that homeopaths work under. You've read a lot of men's names in this book, and it's time for some of the important women practitioners to step forward and be recognized.

I'll show you how to start sorting out the best from the rest, but your judgment and inner sense will serve you in the end. Regardless of who you choose to be your homeopath, stick with the process.

Finding a Qualified Homeopath

Once you have decided to use homeopathic medicines as part of your family's health care, it's time to find the best practitioner for your needs. There are many different kinds of practitioners to choose from. Medical doctors (M.D.s) and osteopathic doctors (O.D.s) who received postgraduate homeopathic training will often have DHT following their names showing board certification as a diplomat in homeotherapeutics. Naturopathic physicians who are board certified through the Homeopathic Academy of Naturopathic Physicians will put DHANP after their names. The designation CCH (Certified in Classical Homeopathy) is for all homeopathic practitioners including chiropractors, veterinarians, acupuncturists, dentists, nurses, physician assistants, and certified nurse midwives.

Now that you've seen the potential cast of characters, I believe the real issues come down to some practical concerns. Find out if the practitioner specializes in homeopathy or doesn't rely on homeopathy a great deal in his practice. How long has he been practicing homeopathy; do you have a friend or personal reference that has been satisfied with his services?

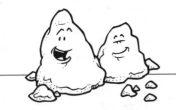

Natural Nuggets

The first step in finding a qualified homeopath can be done through national organizations with high educational standards. Contact The National Center for Homeopathy, The North American Society of Homeopaths, or The Council on Homeopathic Education (all listed in Appendix E, "Homeopathic Schools") for information about a homeopath who fits your needs.

The licensure of a practitioner may have little to do with his homeopathic knowledge. It may, however, help in his management of and familiarity with the specific condition you want treated. If you have a horse, of course, you may want a vet. It's always best to feel satisfied and confident with your choice. During your first visit, do you feel comfortable with this practitioner? After you've had all your questions answered, take a moment to reflect and trust your inner voice to be your guide.

Education and Certification

How do you get to be a homeopath? There are a multitude of training and certification programs both in the United States and overseas. I've included a comprehensive list in Appendix E for your convenience. It's worth mentioning at this time that there are no diplomas or certificates from any school or program that constitute a license to practice homeopathy.

Homeopaths usually serve the public within the boundaries of their existing medical license, whether they be medical doctors, nurses, naturopaths, acupuncturists, or veterinarians. Curiosity and love of learning are essential traits for a good homeopath. A lifetime of learning awaits from conferences, teachers in private practice, and, of course, the patients.

Professional homeopathic organizations have aided the general public and homeopathic practitioners by monitoring the profession and establishing educational guidelines. This will ensure that classical homeopathic medicine is being offered in a responsible, safe, and effective way to the growing numbers of people who wish to choose it as a health-care option.

Women in Homeopathy

History is filled with examples of women being denied their place in business, higher education, voting booths, government, and professional societies. Yet their role in influencing the course of events has become increasingly less covert and more overt. It's about time! The gentle and safe nature of homeopathy attracted the attention of many women who were seeking help with their own health issues and those of their children. The daily observations that a conscientious mother would make are exactly the information that a homeopath uses to find a remedy. I usually ask mothers, "Tell me what's special about your child." Their information is invaluable. Many women learned about homeopathic treatments and administered good care to their families and friends.

The society slowly evolved due to the persistence of women and their advocates, and so did the opportunities for participation in the education and practice of medicine. Slowly, but surely, the tide turned for women in medicine:

➤ **1850:** Female Medical College of Pennsylvania (FMCP) is established, becoming the first medical school for women.

➤ **1867:** Dr. Ann Preston, a member of FMCP, becomes the first woman dean of a U.S. medical school.

➤ **1941:** Hahnemann Medical College first opens enrollment to women.

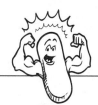

Potent Pellets

The use of homeopathy in the treatment of one person by another may constitute the practice of medicine, depending on the state, which requires a license. Homeopathic medicines are classified as drugs by the FDA; most are over-the-counter, some are prescription only. One must typically be a licensed health-care provider to practice homeopathy in the United States.

Source: The National Center for Homeopathy

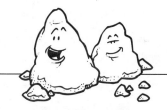

Natural Nuggets

Three states have homeopathic licensing laws: Arizona (1982), Connecticut (1892), and Nevada (1983). M.D.s and D.O.s practicing homeopathy in Arizona or Nevada, and M.D.s practicing in Connecticut must be licensed by the state homeopathic licensing board.

Source: The National Center for Homeopathy

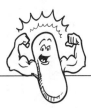

Potent Pellets

Elizabeth Cady Stanton is one of the best-known "lay women" advocates of homeopathy. A religious liberal, health reformer, and major figure in the struggle for women's suffrage and equality, she treated Irish immigrant families working on the Erie Canal. In 1863, she lobbied the New York Legislature and won a charter for New York Medical College and Hospital for Women, a homeopathic institution (Kirschmann, 1997).

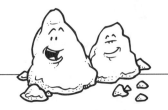

Natural Nuggets

A comprehensive view of women in homeopathy can be found in the November 3, 1997, edition of *The American Homeopath.* This thorough and interesting journal can be obtained from The North American Society of Homeopaths, listed in Appendix E.

➤ **1966:** The School of Health Professions is created from Hahnemann Medical College and Female Medical College of Pennsylvania (formerly FMCP).

The valuable contributions of women in the field of homeopathy continue, as seen by the number of prominent female practitioners and lecturers, researchers, and authors.

Sticking with Homeopathy

Your homeopath may see you for a half hour, perhaps once a month, with the rest of the time being left up to you to carry on the healing work. When you leave the office, you should have a good idea of the treatment plan created by your homeopath. I encourage patients to call if they have any questions or concerns about their progress. A small fear about your condition can grow into a mountain of misconceptions. Usually a two-minute phone call takes care of it all.

I hear patients remark how wonderful it is to feel connected, centered, and have an awareness of their bodies and emotions. They know that when we sit down, I will ask them, "What's been going on since we last met?" They develop skills of self-awareness, patience for observation, and experience the rewards of being part of their own healing. Patients can still get disillusioned. There are many more advertisements on television, newspapers, and tabloids touting the talents and speed of relief for pharmaceutical drugs than there are for homeopathics.

Sometimes people will just quit for a while. Many times they return and are welcomed back. We discuss their reasons for giving up homeopathy and clear up any questions, misconceptions, or expectations that may have led to their frustrations. Good communication with your homeopath is essential for the steady progress that both you and your homeopath desire.

The Least You Need to Know

➤ Finding the right homeopath has been made easier by professional organizations that list their members' location, education, and medical licensure information.

➤ Make sure you are comfortable with your homeopaths and their knowledge of your condition.

➤ Homeopathic education is available to everyone through several national training programs and local study groups.

➤ Women continue to provide valuable insights, guidance, and teaching in the field of homeopathy.

➤ Contact your homeopath if you have any questions or concerns regarding your condition; good communication is an essential part of your healing process.

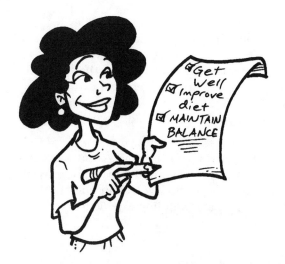

Chapter 26

The Final Touches

In This Chapter

➤ Participate in the pace of your healing

➤ Discover your dynamic potential for healing

➤ The benefits of balance

➤ Learn to experience total freedom

Freedom, peace of mind, and joy are not just for other people: They're for you, too! The benefits are real, and so is the path you take to get there. Will you be turned away easily by the occasionally bumpy terrain, or are you willing to wind your way to the life and inner peace you've dreamed of? Your homeopath, like other trusted professionals and friends, can be a temporary guide, but the journey, the lessons, and yes, the rewards are yours.

This last chapter is chock-full of motivational tidbits to speed you on your way. An enlightened intellect or a more flexible focus may be the result of reading this book. The action steps necessary to successfully stay on the path of purpose and freedom are up to you. Read ahead, and I'll show you a final set of landmarks.

The Evolution of Healing

I often remind patients that healing is not a horse race. There may be preconceived ideas about how much time or effort you believe it will take to achieve your goals. Often people are referred by an enthusiastic friend who experienced a beneficial

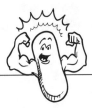

Potent Pellets

Modifiable health risks (the kinds you *can* change!) accounted for more than 25 percent of health-care expenditures in an average year for employers. A breakdown of employees' health risks included high stress (7.9 percent), tobacco use (5.6 percent), being overweight (4.1 percent), and poor experience habits (3.3 percent). Instituting programs to address these health risks would benefit both employees and employers.

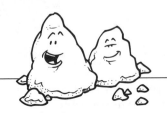

Natural Nuggets

Older men can achieve some of the same benefits in strength improvement as their younger counterparts with regular weight-training exercises. A recent study of men 60 to 75 years of age showed that weight training twice weekly improved their strength by 50 to 84 percent.

Source: onhealth.com

course of treatment with homeopathy. They recount the speedy relief they experienced since they were cared for in our office. You've read some fantastic stories of lightning-fast healing as well as the sure and steady approach of getting better. Your own path to recovery depends on who you are, your medical history, and what you're willing to do to help or hinder the process.

Other healing paths will be in view as you walk, crawl, or sprint down yours. Keep in mind the powers you exercise by choosing to be involved in one of the most illuminating and fulfilling experiences: homeopathic healing.

Lifestyle Matters

Well-prescribed homeopathic remedies assist you in creating a window of opportunity where your body and mind can begin to heal. Think of your illness being completely in your face—like standing too close to a television or movie screen. It's all-encompassing and difficult to get perspective with regard to how you feel and what you can do about it. A remedy can help your body and mind begin to heal while helping you to pull back from the intensity of your complaints. With a new outlook and fresh perspective, the remedy can continue helping so that your good lifestyle choices can make a real difference in your progression.

Exercise has been called a "healthy pleasure" and is one of the single most healthful habits to add to your life. Benefits of exercise include ...

➤ Increased stamina.

➤ Weight loss.

➤ Improved work performance.

➤ Reduced stress and tension.

➤ Better quality of sleep.

➤ Helps prevent diseases such as high blood pressure, cancer, diabetes, and heart disease.

➤ Improved quality of life.

Look at health as a common-sense question. What have I done today that my body will thank me for later? If you are struggling to think of an answer, then you may want to commit to a change, of course.

Your body will begin to give you positive feedback about your healthful choices. The conditions that you have consulted your homeopath on will most often be aided by your participation in the process. By adding more items to the list of "what have I done today to be healthy," you'll increase your chances of a lifestyle that will continue to support you once the homeopath's efforts are no longer needed.

Balance

I suggest using the rule of threes. If you have one particularly stressful day, then give yourself a chance of recovering by allowing two days of low-stress scheduling. The world may not give you a break, but why not make a two-day commitment to handle the way you react to stress more creatively. Enjoy a lunch, call a good friend, or exercise. Blowing off your normal diet of healthful foods for a day of premeditated gorging? Use the next two days to eat only when you're actually hungry, drink plenty of fluids, and eat light, easy-to-digest fruits and vegetables. It can be a balancing act when your body's been ravaged by the conflicts of convenient living.

How much time do you spend goofing off, playing silly games with your children, or volunteering in an organization that could use your help? Getting out of my own cloistered clinic is great for my perspective. When I lend a hand to the elderly, the homeless, or high school kids, I'm always amazed by the diversity of our personal disasters. My problems seem to pale next to the passionate suffering of a teenager whose affections have not been returned. My little efforts seem to benefit others, and the change does me a world of good.

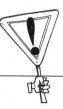

Caution Keeper

The words *all natural* may sometimes mean *all sugar*. High-fructose corn syrup can be just as unhealthy as eating white sugar. Beware! Refined sugars are often camouflaged as corn syrup, fructose, dextrose, dextrin, refined sugar beets, honey, or maple syrup that is not pure, but contains high-fructose corn syrup.

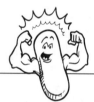

Potent Pellets

A 1998 survey sponsored by the National Sleep Foundation (NSF) found that 40 million Americans suffer from sleep disorders; two out of three people are not getting eight hours of sleep a night, while a third are getting less than six hours.

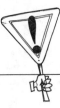

Your homeopath can be a rich resource of ways to help you anchor in your new-found health. As you regain more strength and are able to be proactive in your own care, adding healthful habits to your day sustains your progress. Spend time with the people that really matter to you. Let them know how much they mean to you. Tell a joke, change your wardrobe, do the unexpected that reflects the new choices you are making in your life.

Caution Keeper

That frown could bring you down. A recent study shows that people with heart disease were 40 percent less likely to laugh in humorous situations than those with healthy hearts. The people with heart disease were much less likely to even recognize humor.

Source: Center for Preventative Cardiology at the University of Maryland Medical Center

Freedom!

What would you do with your life if you were free of any physical, mental, or emotional conditions that limit your health? The possibilities are endless! The goal of homeopathy is to help you get as close to that goal as possible. You can always feel better and experience more freedom, even if you still need medications or other therapies to deal with your illnesses.

Being a homeopath allows me the privilege of watching the steady improvement of a person (or whole family) as he frees himself from the conditions that have shaped his life and relationships. How much has your image of yourself been affected and shaped by your disease or diagnosis? Homeopathic philosophy promotes a medicine that at its very core acknowledges the wisdom and unlimited ability of your being.

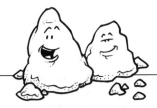

Natural Nuggets

Family reading creates balance and benefits. A recent report correlates family reading with later reading comprehensive and greater school success in children. In 1996, 57 percent of ages 3–5 were read to by family members. That number dropped to 53 percent in 1999. Let's do our part to engage and educate our children.

Source: The National Center for Education Statistics

I hope that this book has given you the courage to step into your own healing destiny. There are ways to incorporate homeopathy into your current healing process. Take the first step. The universe is poised to support your actions.

The Least You Need to Know

➤ Your complete healing depends on your actions to either help or hinder the process.

➤ A well-prescribed homeopathic remedy creates a window of opportunity for self-healing.

➤ Healthy habits like regular exercise, laughter, and good nutrition help sustain benefits of homeopathic care.

➤ Freedom of body, mind, and spirit is the ultimate goal of homeopathy.

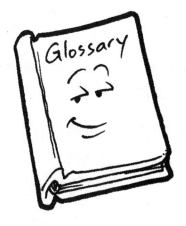

Glossary

cluster theory   Formed when a solution is diluted, placed in water and shaken, as in homeopathic preparations. The water surrounding the solution begins to harden and form crystals or even ice at room temperature.

dilution   Watering down of a substance.

electromagnetic field   The "electromotive force" of water can be measured by putting two identical stainless steel electrodes in water and measuring the potential.

generalized anxiety disorder (GAD)   Excessive daily worry or restlessness about a number of activities or events, lasting for more than six months.

grief   Suffering hardship caused by trouble or sorrow.

Hahnemann, Samuel (1755–1843)   Founder of a new medical system he named homeopathy.

Hering, Constantine (1800–1880)   The founder of American homeopathy.

Hering's direction of cure   According to this theory, as a patient recovers from a disease, the symptoms move from within outward, from above downward, from the center to circumference, and disappear in reverse order of their appearance.

homeopathic provings   Trials conducted with healthy individuals who are given undiluted or lightly diluted doses of an unknown substance until it produces symptoms that are meticulously recorded and collated to form a database of symptoms.

homeopathic remedy   Prepared from plant, animal, or mineral extracts. A substance that, undiluted, can induce a certain group of symptoms in a healthy person, and is capable, in a highly diluted form, of treating similar symptoms in a sick person.

homeopathy   A method of stimulating or provoking the body to defend itself rather than using the usual methods of blocking body responses by drugs.

Kent, James Tyler (1849–1916) Developed homeopathic insight and philosophy and developed a better-organized system of referencing symptoms with homeopathic medicines.

law of similars According to this law, any medicines that are capable of producing disease-like symptoms in a healthy person have the potential to remove similar symptoms occurring in an ill person.

manic depression A condition accompanied by anxiety, intense irritability, or an uncomfortable feeling of being too energetic.

materia medica Medical matters that are the records of the homeopathic provers' symptoms; usually categorized in the same format as the repertory (mind, head, back, abdomen, skin, and so on).

minimum dose Allows a homeopath to give you the smallest possible amount of a remedy that will gently, yet effectively, elicit a reaction from your body's vital force so that healing can begin.

modalities Described as something that holds special attributes or emphasis that marks certain individuals, things, or groups. Modalities typically illustrate when and in what circumstances you feel better or worse during your illness.

night terrors Sudden awakening with inconsolable panic and screaming that usually occur in the first one to three hours of sleep.

panic attacks Sudden episodes of uncontrolled terror described by many people (as if they're having a heart attack, going crazy, or even dying); a serious medical condition that affects twice as many women as men, often beginning in young adulthood between the ages of 15 and 25.

potentize A term coined by Dr. Samuel Hahnemann in the early 1800s; means combining of several dilutions of an original substance via vigorous shaking. The potency of a homeopathic remedy is based on the dilution ratio: the ratio of active substance to inactive base.

repertory Classifies symptoms according to association with different systems such as mind, head, stomach, back, abdomen, and so on.

strange, rare, and peculiar symptoms Unusual sensations or symptoms experienced spontaneously and felt strongly by the patient, which become a core clue to a homeopathic case.

succussion The forceful pounding or vigorous shaking of a liquid dilution against a firm but resilient surface.

vital force The source and sustenance of life; a reliable indicator of how your body is coping with the stresses of disease.

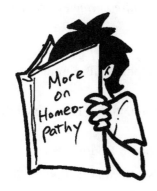

Further Reading

Allen, T.F. *The Encyclopedia of Pure Materia Medica.* New Delhi, India. Jain Publishers Pvt. Limited, 1990.

American Journal of Clinical Nutrition, August 2000.

American Journal of Critical Care Medicine, 2000.

American Journal of Psychiatry, March 2000.

Archives of Diseases in Childhood, Fetal and Neonatal, 2000 Edition.

Bach, Edward. *Heal Thyself: The Bach Flower Remedies; Including Heal Thyself, the Twelve Healers, the Bach Remedies Repertory.* Keats Publishing, 1997.

Balch, James F., and Phyllis A. Balch. *Prescription for Nutritional Healing.* Garden City Park, NY. Avery Publishing Group, 1997.

British Medical Journal 302, Feb. 9, 1991.

Buegel, Dale, Blair Lewis, and Dennis Chernin. *Homeopathic Remedies for Health Professionals and Laypeople.* Himalayan, 1991.

California Journal of Hospital Pharmacy, "Regulation of the Homeopathic Industry." R. Middleton. Dec. 1993.

Castro, Miranda. *The Complete Homeopathy Handbook.* New York. St. Martin's Press, 1991.

———. *Homeopathy for Pregnancy, Birth, and Your Baby's First Year.* St. Martin's Press, 1993.

———. *Homeopathic Guide to Stress.* St. Martin's Press, 1997.

Cummings, Stephen, and Dana Ullman. *Everybody's Guide to Homeopathic Medicines: Safe and Effective Remedies for You and Your Family.* Los Angeles. J.P. Tarcher, 1997.

Curtis, Helena. *Biology.* New York. Worth Publishers, Inc., 1983.

Del Mar, C., Glasziou, P., and M. Hayem. "Are Antibiotics Indicated as Initial Treatment for Children with Acute Otitis Media?" *Alternative Therapies,* Volume 4, Number 5 (1998): 86.

Digestive Diseases and Sciences, June 2000.

Dorland's Pocket Medical Dictionary, 23rd Edition. Philadelphia. W.B. Saunders Company, 1982.

Downey, Paul. *Homeopathy for the Primary Healthcare Team.* Jordan Hill, England. Butterworth-Heinemann, 1997.

Golub, Edward S. *The Limits of Medicine.* New York. Random House. 1994.

Gray, Bill. *Homeopathy: Science or Myth?* Berkeley, CA. North Atlantic Books, 2000.

Guide of Coverage of Complementary and Alternative Medicine, 2000 Edition.

Hahnemann, Samuel. *Organon of the Medical Art.* Edited and annotated by Wenda Brewster O'Reilly. Redmond, WA. Birdcage Books, 1996.

Hamilton, Don. *Homeopathic Care for Cats and Dogs.* Berkeley, CA. North Atlantic Books, 1999.

Henriques, Nicola. *Crossroads to Cure: The Homeopath's Guide to Second Prescription.* St. Helena, CA. Totality Press, 1998.

Homeopathy Today, February 1997.

Infertility and Sterility, July 2000.

Jacobs, Jennifer, article in *Pediatrics,* p. 93; pp. 719–725, 1994.

Jean-Murat, Dr. Carrolle. *Natural Pregnancy.* National Institutes of Health.

Jonas, Wayne B., and Jennifer Jacobs. *Healing with Homeopathy: The Complete Guide.* Warner Books, 1996.

The Journal of Alternative and Complementary Medicine, June 2000.

Journal of the American Medical Association (JAMA), November 24, 1995 & September 2, 2000.

The Journal of Diabetes Care, September 1999.

Journal of Head Trauma and Rehabilitation, p. 14; pp. 521–543, 1999.

Kent, James. *Lectures on Homeopathic Philosophy.* Berkeley, CA. North Atlantic Books, 1979.

Kirschmann, Anne Taylor. "Women and Homeopathy in the 19th Century." *The American Homeopath, 3,* p. 100, 1997.

The Lancet. The Lancet Publishing Co. England, 1997.

Lockie, Andrew. *The Family Guide to Homeopathy.* New York. Prentice-Hall, 1991.

McCabe, Vinton. *Practical Homeopathy*. New York. Griffin Trade, 2000.

Merck Manual, 17th Edition. Whitehouse Station, NJ. Merck Research Laboratories, 1999.

Morrison, Roger, M.D. *Desktop Guide to Keynotes and Confirmatory Symptoms*. Albany, CA. Hahnemann Clinic Publishing, 1993.

Moskowitz, Richard, M.D. *Homeopathic Medicines for Pregnancy and Childbirth*. Berkeley, CA. North Atlantic Books, 1992.

New England Journal of Medicine, October 8, 2000.

O'Reilly, Wenda Brewster, editor and translator. *Organon of the Medical Art*. Redmond, WA. Birdcage Books, 1996.

Pawlak, Dr. Laura. *Estrogen Dilemmas*. Redondo Beach, CA. Fresh Graphics, 1996.

PDR for Herbal Medicines, 2nd Edition. Montvale, NJ. Medical Economics Company, 2000.

Psychosomatic Medicine, July/August 2000. Centers for Disease Control and Prevention.

Reichenberg-Ullman, Judyth. *Prozac-Free: Homeopathic Medicine for Depression, Anxiety, and Other Mental and Emotional Problems*. Rocklin, CA. Prima Publishing, 1999.

————. *Whole Woman Homeopathy: The Comprehensive Guide to Treating PMS, Menopause, Cystitis, and Other Problems—Naturally and Effectively*. Rocklin, CA. Prima Publishing, 2000.

The Robert Wood Johnson Foundation's 1999 Annual Report.

Sankaran, Rajan. *The Spirit of Homeopathy*. Bombay, India. Homeopathic Medical Publishers, 1991.

————. *The Substance of Homeopathy*. Bombay, India. Homeopathic Medical Publishers, 1994.

Sault, David. *A Modern Guide and Index to the Mental Rubrics of Kent's Repertory*. Haarlem, Holland. Merlyn Publishers, 1992.

Scholten, Jan. *Homeopathy and the Elements*. Utrecht, The Netherlands. Stichting Alonnissos, 1996.

Sher, Jeremy. *The Dynamics and Methodology of Homoeopathic Provings*. West Malvern, England. Dynamis Books, 1994.

————. *The Proving of Chocolate*. West Malvern, England. Dynamis Books, 1999.

Somonides. *An Essay on Women*. 6th century B.C.E.

The State of Healthcare in America, 1998.

Stoler, Diane. *Coping with Mild Traumatic Brain Injury*. Garden City Park, NY. Avery Publishing Group, 1998.

Ullman, Dana. *Homeopathic Medicine for Children and Infants*. New York. J.P. Tarcher/ Putnam, 1992.

Ullman, Robert, and Judyth Reichnberg-Ullman. *Rage-Free Kids: Homeopathic Medicine for Defiant, Aggressive, and Violent Children*. Rocklin, CA. Prima Publishing, 1999.

————. *Homeopathic Self-Care: The Quick and Easy Guide for the Whole Family*. Rocklin, CA. Prima Publishing, 1997.

Vithoulkas, George. *Science of Homeopathy*. New York. Grove Press, 1980.

Weil, Andrew. *Natural Health, Natural Medicine: A Comprehensive Manual for Wellness and Self-Care*. Oxfordshire, Great Britain. Houghton Mifflin Company, 1998.

Wessell, Norman, and Janet Hopson. *Biology*. New York. Random House, Inc., 1988.

Yasgur, Jay. *A Dictionary of Homeopathy Medical Terminology*. Greenville, PA. Van Hoy Publishers, 1990.

Resources

Homeopathic Software

Software tools for homeopathic practitioners including MacRepertory and ReferenceWorks.

Kent Homeopathic Associates
710 Mission Avenue
San Rafael, CA 94901
415-457-0678
1-877-YES-KENT
Fax: 415-457-0688
E-mail: kah@igc.org
www.kenthomeopathic.com

Hahnemann Laboratories
1940 Fourth Street
San Rafael, CA 94901
www.hahnemannlabs.com

Web Sites

www.biausa.org, Brain Injury Association (BIA), 202-296-6443

www.caisinet/nario/hirhtml, *Head Injury Resource Guide* for people with head injuries and their families

www.homeopathy.org

www.onhealth.com

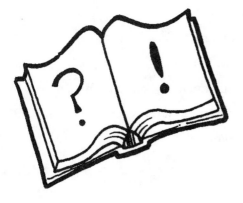

Homeopathic Pharmacy Terminology

Homeopathics are prepared with many of the standard pharmaceutical processes: the Roman numerals that indicate the number of dilutions or potentization are often confusing. This quick reference, provided by Hahnemann Laboratories, Inc., is a guide to understanding the solution to the dilution.

potentization   Process of preparing homeopathic remedies.

dynamization   Process of preparing homeopathic remedies.

attenuation   Process of preparing homeopathic remedies.

succussion	Forceful pounding of vial against a book.
dilution	Decreasing concentration of raw material.
Korsakovian	Single-vial preparation method.
Hahnemannian	Many-vial preparation method.
fluxion	Flowing water method of potentization.
continuous fluxion	Continuous flowing water method.
maceration	Soaking in alcohol.
tincture	Alcoholic liquid.
mother tincture	Source alcoholic liquid.
centesimal	One to 100 (1:100).
decimal	One to 10 (1:10).
quinquagentessimal	One to 50,000 (1:50,000).
LM	Quinquagentessimal dilution process.
Q	Quinquagentessimal dilution process.

X	Decimal dilution process.
C	Centesimal dilution process.
K	Korsakovian dilution process.
CH	Centesimal Hahnemannian dilution process.
CK	Centesimal Korsakovian dilution process.
D	Decimal dilution process.
M	1,000c.
1M	1,000c.
10M	10,000c.
XM	10,000c.
50M	50,000c.
LM	50,000c (technically correct but dangerous).
CM	100,000c.
MM	1,000,000c.
HPUS	*Homeopathic Pharmacopoeia of the U.S.*
AAHP	American Association of Homeopathic Pharmacists.
FDA	Food and Drug Administration.
OTC	Over the counter.
proactive	Inducing purchase.
reactive	Responding to request.
LD50	Lethal dose to 50 percent of the population.

Source: Hahnemann Laboratories, Inc. For more information visit www.hahnemannlabs.com.

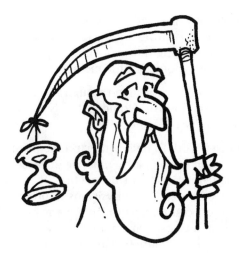

A Brief History of Homeopathy

The story of homeopathy in this country reads like the script for a TV soap opera. Here's a look at the highlights of the pioneers' triumphs, the obstacles, challenges, political intrigue, and conspiracies, followed by a resurgence of homeopathy that still strongly continues.

(Note: This history was compiled and written by The Institute of Classical Homeopathy and contains a few of my additions.)

The roots of homeopathic philosophy date from fourth-century B.C.E. Greek and other ancient and medieval medical texts. Homeopathy is a complete system of healing discovered by Dr. Samuel Hahnemann in 1796, which recognizes that all life is sustained by a vital force. Since then it has been practiced successfully worldwide, and in North America for more than 170 years. Homeopathy was the first medical system to recognize the importance of hygiene and diet in maintaining health, and its practitioners were the first to carry out scientific drug trials. In the United States between 1820 and 1910, two medical traditions and theories coexisted to heal the sick: homeopathy, which implements the law of similiars, and allopathy, which implements the law of opposites (see Chapter 24, "Who's Driving Your Health Bus?").

1820–1830: First homeopaths to practice in the United States were European M.D.s and pupils of Dr. Samuel Hahnemann.

1835: Founding of first American medical school of homeopathy by Dr. Constantine Hering, graduate of Würzburg University, Hahnemann's pupil.

1842: New York Medical Society condemns homeopathy; refuses practice license to homeopathic doctors.

1843: Hahnemann dies in Paris.

1844: Establishment of the first U.S. National Medical Association—American Institute of Homeopathy. Its charter is to license homeopathic physicians; maintain standards of education and practice; and serve as a clearing house of "provings" (drug trials) of North American native plants and other new homeopathic medicines.

1845–1910: Twenty-two homeopathic medical schools established throughout the United States, and 15,000 homeopathic practitioners flourish. Homeopathy is considered more successful, economical, and patient friendly than allopathy.

1846: A national medical convention meets in New York to review the "problem" of homeopathy. Delegates conclude the great success of homeopathy must be due solely to allopathic physician's bad marketing and public relations. At this meeting, the American Medical Association (AMA) was founded as a guild of physicians to protect the business interests of its members, and as a direct counterpart to the American Institute of Homeopathy. A well-organized campaign to ostracize homeopathy and dominate the practice of medicine in the United States is launched and continues today.

1849: Cholera epidemic of "The U.S. South." Using homeopathically prepared medicine, homeopaths are more successful than allopaths in treating the sick.

1849: Arrival in California of the "forty-niner" homeopaths at the gold rush.

1850–1900: Little or no federal/state control over medical education exists.

1855: AMA condemns mixing homeopathy with standard medical practice; withholds membership from any state and local medical organizations to which homeopaths belong.

1856: AMA bans any discussion of homeopathic medical theory in its journals and expels doctors who consult with homeopaths; allopaths married to homeopaths are also expelled.

1860–1865: American Civil War.

1860: Birth of the American pharmaceutical industry manufacturing traditional medicines.

1866: Drug companies begin to expand their influence and territory. Patent medicine industry evolves.

1867: Pacific Homeopathic Medical Society of California founded.

1877: Founding of California State Homeopathic Medical Association.

1900: Drug companies and AMA doctors become allies against homeopaths.

1903: AMA claims nonsectarianism, lures banned homeopaths to rejoin, and takes over homeopathic medical schools. Homeopathic medical education is thus undermined and the homeopathic movement begins to weaken.

1910: American Institute of Homeopathy attempts to strengthen its weakened position, but individual homeopaths are not interested in political activism.

1918: Seven homeopathic medical schools remain in existence.

1924: The formation of the American Foundation for Homeopathy (AFH). Formed by a group of 12 physicians and laypeople, the AFH was founded to provide homeopathic education to physicians as a postgraduate course, and to provide general education to laypeople.

1938: The U.S. Food and Drug Administration (FDA) founded. Homeopathic remedies are included in FDA legislation because they were in the *Homeopathic Pharmacopoeia*. It, along with the *U.S. Pharmacopoeia*, was listed as one of the two official drug manuals. AMA continues to dominate new "health industry."

1940s: Last students from U.S. homeopathic medical schools graduate. (The majority of the physicians who kept homeopathy alive from 1930 to 1970 were trained by the AFH.)

1948: Hahnemann Medical College of Philadelphia (founded by Hering) survives and graduates homeopaths through the early 1940s, but is eventually influenced by allopathy. Homeopathy is dropped as a mandatory course in 1948.

1960: Decline of American homeopathy due to death of remaining practitioners, lack of interest, and lack of homeopathic training courses.

1970: Birth of self-help health era; resurgence of interest in homeopathy begins. Most of those involved in the resurgence received their training from the AFH.

1974: The National Center for Homeopathy (NCH) begins administration of the AFH school.

1978: Conference of U.S. homeopaths convenes at California Academy of Sciences. Launch of International Foundation of Homeopathy (IFH), to raise standards of homeopathic practice and promote homeopathy throughout North America and the world.

1980–1990s: Expansion of homeopathic education and training courses. Some 3,000 homeopaths practice.

1999: The NCH celebrates its 25th anniversary and continues to be instrumental in keeping homeopathy alive in the United States.

2000–present: Cost of allopathic conventional medicine is skyrocketing. Managed health care (HMO) prevails. Millions of Americans cannot afford health insurance. To avoid high-cost hospitalization fees, HMOs are wisely conducting various cost-benefit analyses of alternative (to allopathic) healing systems. Where efficacy and cost-efficiency are proved, certain alternative healing systems are offered by these pioneering health plans with an eye on the significance of preventative medicine. To regain control of their health, more and more Americans spend billions of dollars annually on out-of-pocket/over-the-counter homeopathic and other alternative medicines and therapies. Public demand grows for high-quality homeopathic care from expertly trained, highly skilled Hahnemannian homeopaths. The AMA continues to discipline members practicing homeopathy and other alternative therapies.

Founding of the national U.S. Citizens for Health Freedom Organization, established to defend the right of individuals to practice and receive medicine of their choice.

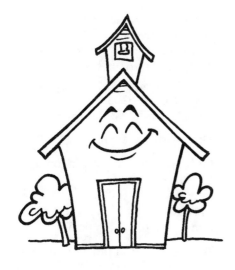

Homeopathic Schools

Schools with an asterisk (*) preceding the name offer programs currently applying for accreditation. All others are accredited programs.

Postgraduate Courses

A professional health-care license is required. Postgraduate and graduate programs are in a part-time, weekend format unless part of a doctor of naturopathy (N.D.) program or otherwise noted.

Canadian Academy of Homeopathy
3044 Bloor St. West, Suite 203
Toronto, ON M8X 1C4
416-503-4003
Fax: 416-503-2799

Three-year program; not currently beginning a new class.

Hahnemann College of Homeopathy
80 Nicholl Ave.
Pt. Richmond, CA 94801
510-232-2079
Fax: 510-512-9044
E-mail: hahnemann@ibc.apc.org

Four-year program.

*Homeopathic College of Canada
280 Eglinton Ave. East
Toronto, ON M4P 1L4
416-481-8816
Fax: 416-481-4444
E-mail: info@homeopath.org

Three-year program; part-time.

*Homeopathy for the Primary Care Provider
Ted Chapman, M.D.
91 Cornell St.
Newton Lower Falls, MA 02162-1320
617-244-8780

Forty-hour program.

*International College of
Homeopathy
8306 Wilshire Blvd. #728
Beverly Hills, CA 90211
310-645-0443
Fax: 310-645-1914

Two-year program.

**National Center for Homeopathy
Summer School**
801 N. Fiarfax St., Suite 306
Alexandria, VA 22314-1757
703-548-7790
Fax: 703-548-7792
E-mail: info@homeopathic.org

*New England School of
Homeopathy
356 Middle St.
Amherst, MA 01002
413-256-5949
Fax: 413-256-6223
E-mail: herscu@nesh.com

Three-year program.

*Teleosis School of Homeopathy
61 W. 62nd St.
New York, NY 10023
212-707-8481
E-mail: teleosis@igc.apc.org

Two-year clinical program; two-year
certificate program with additional
two years of clinical training.

Graduate Courses

The following programs are open to licensed and unlicensed persons.

*Bastyr University
14500 Juanita Dr. N.E.
Bothell, WA 98011
206-823-1300
www.bastyr.edu

396 hours part of N.D. program.

***Caduceus Institute of Classical
Homeopathy**
516 Caledonia St.
Santa Cruz, CA 95062
1-800-396-9778 or 831-466-3516
E-mail: homeoUSA@aol.com
www.homeopathyhome.com/caduceus

Two hundred sixteen hours over three years.

***Canadian College of Naturopathic
Medicine**
PO Box 2431, 18th Floor
Toronto, ON M4P 1E4
416-486-8584
Fax: 416-484-6821
E-mail: info@ccnm.edu
www.ccnm.edu

Two hundred five hours, part of N.D. program.

***Colorado Institute for Classical
Homeopathy**
2299 Pearl St., Suite 401
Boulder, CO 80302
303-440-3717
Fax: 303-442-6852
E-mail: bseideneck@ aol.com

Two-year program, clinical in
year two.

*Curentur University
5519 South Centinela Ave.
Los Angeles, CA 90066
310-448-1700
Fax: 310-448-1703
E-mail: dean@curentur.org

Six hundred and seventy-five
classroom hours.

*The Homeopathic College
411 Andrews Rd.
University Office, Park Suite 230
Durham, NC 27705
919-286-0500
1-800-218-7733

Four-year program.

*The Institute of Natural Health Sciences
43000 Nine Mile Rd.
Novi, MI 48375
248-473-5458
Fax: 248-473-8141

240 classroom hours plus 100 hours of independent study.

*National Center for Homeopathy
801 North Fairfax, Suite 306
Alexandria, VA 22314
703-548-7790
www.homeopathic.org

Summer school.

National College of Naturopathic Medicine
049 SW Porter St.
Portland, OR 97201
503-499-4343
Fax: 503-499-0022

Lecture and clinical hours, part of N.D. program.

*New England School of Homeopathy
356 Middle St.
Amherst, MA 01002
413-256-5949
Fax: 413-256-6223
E-mail: herscu@nesh.com

Three-year program.

*Northwestern Academy of Homeopathy
10700 Old County Club Rd. 15
Minneapolis, MN 55441
612-794-6445
www.homeopathicschool.org

Three-year program, clinical in third year.

*Pacific Academy of Homeopathic Medicine
1199 Sanchez St.
San Francisco, CA 94114
415-458-8238
Fax: 415-695-8220
E-mail: Pahm@slip.net

Two-year program with clinical, third year optional.

*The School of Homeopathy, New York
964 3rd Ave., 8th Floor
New York, NY 10155-0003
212-570-2576
Fax: 212-758-4079
E-mail: kathy@homeopathyschool.com

Four-year program with clinical.

Toronto School of Homeopathic Medicine
17 Yorkvillle Ave., Suite 200
Toronto, ON M4W 1L1
1-800-572-6001
Fax: 416-966-1724
E-mail: Info@homeopathycanada.com
www.homeopathycanada.com

Three-year program, with clinical training.

*Vancouver Homeopathic Academy
PO Box 34095, Station D
Vancouver, BC V671G8
604-739-4633

Three-year program.

Correspondence Courses (Open to licensed and unlicensed students.)

The British Institute of Homeopathy
520 Washington Blvd., Suite 5109
Marina Del Rey, CA 90292
310-577-2235

Canadian Academy of Homeopathy
1173 Blvd. du Mont Royal
Outremont, PQ H2V 2H6
514-279-6629

Living Water School of Homeopathy
11802 Willow Valley Rd.
Nevada City, CA 95959
530-265-9464

*The School of Homeopathy, Devon, England
82 East Pearl St.
New Haven, CT 06513
203-624-8783 phone/fax

Todd Rowe, M.D.
1118 E. Missouri, Suite A1
Phoenix, AZ 85014
602-439-1589

Episodic Seminars

Althea Homeopathics
1217 West Howe
Seattle, WA 98119
206-284-5320

American Institute of Homeopathy
23200 Edmonds Way, Suite A.
Edmonds, WA 98026
206-542-5595

Dynamis School
c/o Josett Polzella, Administrator
40 Dancing Rock Rd.
Garrison, NY 10524
914-734-9347

Homeopathic Academy of Naturopathic Physicians
12132 S.E. Foster Pl.
Portland, OR 97266
503-761-3298

Murray Feldman & Kim Boutilier
PO Box 34095, Station D
Vancouver, BC V6J4M1
604-708-9387

National Center for Homeopathy
801 North Fairfax St., Suite 306
Alexandria, VA 22314
703-438-7790

Naturally Divine, Inc.
1706 Hall Dr.
Tallahassee, FL 32303
850-386-6970

New England Homeopathic Academy
24 Minot Ave.
Acton, MA 12720
508-635-0605

North American Network of Homeopathic Educators (Teleosis Homeopathic Educators)
3 Main St.
Chatham, NY 12037
518-592-7975

Ohio Homeopathic Medical Society
3531 Longwood Dr.
Medina, OH 44256
330-239-2762

Texas Society of Homeopathy
1111 Highway 6, Suite 150
Sugar Land, TX 77478
281-494-3460

Index

311

Q–R

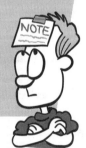